Drug Calculations for Nurses

Context for Practice

Kerri Wright

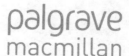

First published 2011 by
PALGRAVE MACMILLAN

Palgrave Macmillan in the UK is an imprint of Macmillan Publishers Limited, registered in England, company number 785998, of Houndmills, Basingstoke, Hampshire RG21 6XS.

Palgrave Macmillan in the US is a division of St Martin's Press LLC, 175 Fifth Avenue, New York, NY 10010.

Palgrave Macmillan is the global academic imprint of the above companies and has companies and representatives throughout the world.

Palgrave® and Macmillan® are registered trademarks in the United States, the United Kingdom, Europe and other countries.

ISBN: 978–0–230–23161–0

This book is printed on paper suitable for recycling and made from fully managed and sustained forest sources. Logging, pulping and manufacturing processes are expected to conform to the environmental regulations of the country of origin.

A catalogue record for this book is available from the British Library.

10 9 8 7 6 5 4 3 2 1
20 19 18 17 16 15 14 13 12 11

Printed in China

Contents

List of Figures and Boxes

Figures

Boxes

Acknowledgements

I would like to thank the following people for their help with reading and checking through early drafts of this book; Cathy Maylin, Anita Lutchman, Terry Ferns and Philip Marini. I would also like to thank all my colleagues at University of Greenwich who have readily given their time to help me in my research on this topic and the students who have been enthusiastic recipients of my teaching and ideas and have continually inspired me to rethink and refine my thoughts. Finally, I'd like to thank Professor Liz Meerabeau who has been a constant encouragement and believer in my work on drug calculations, Pat Williams for her love and compassion and Kate Llewellyn, Project Editor, who has been a patient and thoughtful motivator throughout this project. However, my acknowledgements would not be complete without heartfelt thanks to my partner Joanna and our daughter Bethany; to them the thanks are for everything.

Introduction

Welcome to this friendly and informal approach to drug calculations. I know that maths causes lots of anxiety in people and you may be coming to this book with a heavy heart thinking that you cannot do maths. If you are, you are not alone in these thoughts. I have taught drug calculations to numerous qualified nurses and student nurses and many have stated that they cannot do maths and bring a great deal of anxiety to the sessions. Some of this anxiety is purely related to maths and our beliefs about maths. Some of you may believe that you cannot do maths because of experiences during your formal schooling and have memories of those lessons that still affect your beliefs about maths now. Some student nurses can remember being shouted at by teachers, told to stand in a corner for not getting an answer right or severely punished for producing the wrong answers. With these experiences and memories, it really is no wonder that the thought of doing maths again can cause anxiety!

Although this is a controversial thing to say, I will say it anyway. When you are in clinical practice and solving drug calculations, you are not doing 'maths'. You are nursing. Yes, it is true that you need a basic understanding of numeracy to solve drug calculations and can benefit from knowing how to do basic arithmetic operations such as division and multiplication, but essentially you are performing a nursing skill, not a maths skill. If we put the greatest mathematician into clinical practice and asked them to solve some of the drug dosages you calculate every day in your practice, they would struggle and possibly not be able to do this. Why? Because they have not got your clinical knowledge and skills, which place the drug calculations into a context and allow them to be understood and thus solved. You cannot solve drug calculations with maths alone. Your clinical skills are essential in making sense of the calculations you are solving and applying these to an individual patient's care. So do take some heart that we are not doing 'maths' but are doing 'nursing'.

However, we have to accept that you cannot solve drug calculations without some knowledge and understanding of numeracy. Numeracy is basically an understanding of numbers. You will all have sufficient understanding of numbers in order to function in life. You wouldn't be able to go shopping, pay the bills, and drive a car, for example, if you didn't understand numbers. Numeracy is knowing what numbers are and how they relate to each other, for example that 4 is bigger than 1 and 100 is ten times bigger than 10. Numeracy is often also described as the ability to use the four basic arithmetic functions of addition, subtraction, multiplication and division. This is where things get a little complicated. Understanding and applying the four basic functions just mentioned is commonplace in everyday life. You know that you will need to divide a pizza into eight pieces if you have eight people for dinner and that you will need to halve the ingredients for a cake if you only want to make half the size. We do all these things without thinking about it. The difference comes when we translate this everyday mathematics into formal mathematical language.

Most people would probably not think that dividing our bills into monthly instalments is mathematics and believe that mathematics involves formal operations that they remember from school such as long division, long multiplication, multiplication of fractions, for example. Often school or formal mathematics involves numbers alone and doesn't always give you a context. For example, a bill of £400 to be paid over 5 months would be £400 divided by 5 months and would mean you would need to pay £80 a month. In mathematical notation this might be:

$5\overline{)400}$ or 400 ÷ 5 or $\dfrac{400}{5}$

Without the context of the bill, this can seem baffling. There is a danger therefore that the arithmetic operation doesn't actually make much sense on its own and you are purely manipulating numbers. For example, look at the following arithmetic calculation:

$\dfrac{1000}{500} \times 1 =$

You may be able to work this out because you recognise the numbers in this calculation. Consider, though, the problem that your patient has been prescribed 1000mg and you need to work out how many 500mg tablets you should administer to give 1000mg. With this problem, depending on the amount of nursing experience you have had to date, you are more likely to be able to visualise that you will need two tablets to make up the dose of 1000mg:

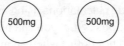

This is very different from the arithmetic notation above, but leads to the same answer.

Nurses are not alone in being able to solve number-based problems in clinical practice, but finding this harder when the same problems are represented in mathematical notation. This difficulty has been highlighted in a number of workplaces where researchers have observed workers carrying out quite complex calculations within their work environment, but then struggling when sat down in a classroom and asked to solve the same problems in a written form using mathematical notation (Nunes et al., 1993).

I am not saying that you do not need arithmetic operations and mathematical knowledge in order to solve drug calculations; these are useful skills to have. However, you can solve most drug calculations through using your everyday numeracy knowledge. To solve calculations in this way, though, you need to be out in clinical practice practising drug calculations as they appear in reality. This helps you to understand exactly what the problem is asking you and helps you to think logically and clearly about how the problem can be solved and whether the answer obtained makes sense. What can happen if too much focus is placed on arithmetic operations such as long division or using a formula is that these procedures are latched onto and what the question is actually asking is neglected. Neglecting the meaning of the question is dangerous. Answers are arrived at blindly and dosages administered that, if the nurses had stopped and thought about it logically, they would know did not make sense.

To illustrate this point, I will give you an example from practice. Say you need to administer 50mg of a drug to your patient. When you go to the stock cupboard the ampoules available each contain 100mg. This means that in every ampoule there is 100mg. Now think logically. If you need to give 50mg and the ampoules each contain 100mg, how much of the ampoule would you administer? If you have got hung up on this, thinking 'agh this is a drug calculation!' I will put it in a different context. You want to cook a small cake. You need 50 grams of butter. The packet of butter you have weighs 100 grams. How much of the butter would you use? I am hoping that now you will have got the answer of half an ampoule and half the butter packet for these problems. You have used your logic to work this out. What I have seen happening in taught calculation sessions is students entering 50 divided 100 into their calculator and obtaining the answer 0.5, but then having no idea at all what this means in relation to practice, that is, what do they do with this information? What do they actually administer?

The danger of practising drug calculations using mathematical formulas and always using written questions is that you can become cut off from the realities of clinical practice and not notice when an answer is illogical clinically or just downright bizarre. One of the problems with this is that nurse educators set questions where the 'right' solution for the question would never be the 'right' dose to give in clinical practice. If you get too adapted to this, then when it comes to clinical practice you can become immune to the triggers that highlight that your solution isn't logical or the usual dose for that drug. I had an example of this during a drug calculation assessment session with qualified nurses. I had clearly informed all the nurses that the questions were based on real doses and so their answers would reflect the reality in clinical practice. Despite this, one answer, given by a very experienced nurse, was '40 tablets'! Once this was highlighted to the nurse she was able to see immediately that this wasn't a dose you would ever administer and checked her work. This highlights that focusing solely on drug calculations in a classroom devoid of clinical experience can be dangerous. To combat this:

1. If you are a student nurse, try to involve yourself in drug administration and practising calculations in clinical practice as much as you can so that you understand what you are actually trying to calculate and get used to the types of calculations and dosages usually administered.

2. If you are already an experienced nurse, then try to imagine what you are physically doing as you solve written drug calculations to help you make the link between the written description and the realities of practice.

3. If you are a nurse educator or involved in teaching calculation skills to nurses, please make sure that your written questions reflect dosages used for drugs in practice so that nurses can use their clinical knowledge to make sense of the questions and, more importantly, use this as a checker for the solution they have obtained. The ideal would be to teach in a clinical environment with the standard equipment available to make this as 'real' as possible.

So what am I saying? I am very strongly saying that you must understand what the drug calculation problem is asking you before trying to solve it. This understanding allows you to have a mental picture in your head of what it is exactly you are trying to work out and how you are going to do this. Not only does this help you to plan and solve your calculation problem but, as the example above illustrates, it will help you to 'know' whether your solution makes sense too. So making sure that you understand what the problem is asking you is one of the most important things you must do to solve calculations effectively and safely. A clear mental picture will guide your planning, solving and examining of the solution you arrive at. Without a clear understanding you are more at risk of making errors and, more worryingly, not even noticing that you have made an error. I shall give you another example to illustrate this. Your patient has been prescribed 20mg oramorph. The suspension available contains 10mg in every 5ml. See illustration below:

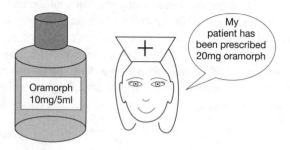

A nurse calculates that they need to administer 2.5ml. Is this answer correct? Apart from calculating the answer for yourself, how do you know just by examining exactly what the question is asking that this solution is wrong? Have a look at the box below to see if your explanation is similar to mine.

Box i   Sample solution

The available drug strength is 10mg in 5ml. This means that every time you give 5ml of this elixir you administer 10mg. Your patient needs 20mg so you need more than 10mg. You will need to administer more than 5ml. You should be able to see that the amount the nurse has decided to administer is less than 5ml, so must logically be incorrect. The nurse should administer 10ml.

Don't worry too much if you are not quite clear about this, we will go over it in more detail later on, where I hope it will make more sense.

● Summary of the Book

In this book I have tried to relate the calculations and explanations to practice so that you are always encouraged to think about what it is you are doing in clinical practice. Ultimately your goal is to be able to calculate drug dosages and rates in a clinical environment so I am always trying to encourage you to think about what you are doing clinically, what your answer represents and what you are now going to do with your answer. It is no good successfully calculating your solution to a calculation as 4, but then not knowing what to do with this! I was struck by this difficulty during a calculation practice session with student nurses. After about an hour of calculating drip rates for infusion bags with the students and their practising this, a very bright student, who had got all the answers right, asked me what the numbers in the answers meant and what she was supposed to do with them! I had forgotten to relate the drip rate to clinical practice and how you apply the answer!

One of the big practical difficulties between calculating a dosage from a written question and doing it in clinical practice is the way that you would obtain the information required to calculate the question. In written calculation questions the information you need is stated for you and more often than not the questions are written in a certain format so that you can actually 'learn' how to solve them without fully understanding what you are actually doing clinically. In clinical practice you have to physically seek out the information required by checking on the medicine chart and going to the patient's locker or drug cupboard to obtain information about the strength of drugs available. It is very difficult to replicate this process in a written book! However, I have attempted to do this by using medicine administration charts and pictures of drug boxes or ampoules to get you used to extracting the information you require. This is obviously still easier than clinical practice where you have to select the right drug medicine administration chart for the patient involved and the right medication from a selection of many in the drug cupboard, but it is a start and hopefully will help you get used to the process involved and feel a bit more 'real'.

Throughout the book you will find sections on 'tips for learning' where I give some thoughts and ideas that could help you to become more confident or adept at working out specific calculations as well as points to bear in mind when you are administering this dose to a patient. As I am also a great believer in seeing the whole context of a calculation and that it is part of the drug administration process, I have also included some general advice related to drug administration in the 'tips for learning' and 'clinical context' boxes as you go though the different calculations.

Along these lines, I've also added some 'Warning!' boxes to remind you to take care on particular calculations or other areas of practice related to the calculation where errors could occur.

I have also included some sections called 'maths explained'. These sections give a brief explanation of the actual mathematics that underpins the methods I am explaining. On occasions, though, these sections will direct you to specific points within Chapter 4 which covers the numeracy required for clinical calculations and drug calculation assessments.

In **Chapter 1**, I have set the clinical context for medication administration and have outlined the different units of measurement for medicine strengths, the different types of medication and different routes by which these can be administered. The calculations I cover in this chapter are converting between units of measurement, calculating dosages prescribed according to patients' weights and calculations dosages prescribed as a daily amount. These skills are the foundations for all other medication calculations and will be built upon in the following chapters.

Chapter 2 will continue with calculating medicine dosages expressed as weight and volume strengths and **Chapter 3** covers calculations involving continuous infusions including syringe drivers. Although you do not have to start at Chapter 1 and work your way to the end of Chapter 3, the calculations do slowly increase in difficulty and build on skills learnt in previous chapters. Therefore I would advise you to be sure you understand the calculating skills in each chapter before you move on.

Chapter 4 gives you an opportunity to practise some specific numeracy skills and apply these to drug calculations. You may wish to do start with this chapter first. It begins with a short maths test to assess your numeracy skills. This will help you to reflect upon which areas of your numeracy and maths you may need to work on. If you find you do need some of your maths skills brushing up, then this chapter will help by giving you a basic reminder of the arithmetic you will need for drug calculations.

Finally, **Chapter 5** offers specific assessments for Chapters 1–3 and also ones for particular clinical contexts. You can use these to simply test your understanding or as practice tests for formal written drug calculation tests.

● And Finally ...

As you may have realised by now, I am a firm believer that calculations need to be carried out within the clinical context and that the skills of calculating doses here are very different from the skills required to solve a written drug calculation assessment.

However, I am also a realist and am aware that despite my belief and evidence to support this (Wright, 2009, 2008, 2007), written drug calculation assessments are still being used as a measure of nurses' and student nurses' competency at drug calculations – which is why I have included a whole chapter on written drug calculation tests (Chapter 5).

To help prepare you, I have also included some calculations which I know are often asked in drug calculation tests and which you would not normally need to calculate in clinical practice. In the future, perhaps all calculation skills will be tested within the clinical environment and within the wider context of drug administration. For now, though, even as I am challenging this, I still need to ensure that you are equipped for all calculations skills assessments you may be given!

Despite this, I cannot stress enough to you the importance of your taking the skills and ideas learnt in this book and practising and applying them to your drug administrations in clinical practice.

All that remains is for me to wish you well on your journey through this calculation guide and hope that I prove to be an amicable, supportive and patient companion to you. So when you are ready, let us begin ...

● References

Nunes, T., Schliemann, A. and Carraher, D. (1993) *Street Mathematics and School Mathematics Learning and Doing: Social, Cognitive and Computational Perspectives* (Cambridge: Cambridge University Press).

Wright, K. (2007) 'Student nurses need more than maths to improve their drug calculating skills', *Nurse Education Today* 25(6): 430–6.

Wright, K. (2008) 'Drug calculations part 1: a critique of the formula used by nurses', *Nursing Standard* 22(36): 40–3.

Wright, K. (2009) 'The assessment and development of drug calculations skills in nurse education – a critical debate', *Nurse Education Today* 29(5): 544–8.

List of Abbreviations

BMI	body mass index
BNF	*British National Formulary*
bpm	beats per minute
BSA	body surface area
COPD	chronic obstructive pulmonary disease
dpm	drips/drops per minute
g	gram
ICU	intensive care unit
IM	intramuscular
ITU	intensive therapy/treatment unit
IU	international units
IV	intravenously
kg	kilogram
L	litre
mcg	microgram
mg	milligram
ml	millilitre
mmol	millimole
NG	naso gastro tube
NMC	Nursing and Midwifery Council
PCA	patient controlled analgesia
PEG	percutaneous endoscopic gastrostomy tube
SC or s/c	subcutaneously
SIU	standardised international units
U	units

Part I

Drug calculations in context

1 Back to Basics! Calculating and understanding simple medicine dosages

66 *Setting the scene and laying the foundations* 99

● Units of Measurement

I am going to go right back to very basics to help you understand units of measurement. The amount of drug that is prescribed for a patient is specific according to their clinical condition, their weight and the therapeutic effect of that drug. In order to ensure that this amount is administered, we need to be able to measure the drug. This is similar to when you are baking a cake; you need to have specific amounts of each ingredient, for example flour or eggs. Most drugs are measured according to their weight or their volume, or their weight and volume together.

The main units of measurement for weight used in clinical practice are kilograms, grams, milligrams, micrograms and nanograms (see Box 1). The main units of measurement for volume are litres and millilitres (see Box 1).

Box 1   Common measurements used in drug dosages, with abbreviations

Measurement	Abbreviation	Size order	Measurement	Abbreviation
Grams	g	Decreasing in size	Litres	L
Milligrams	mg		Millilitres	ml
Micrograms	mcg			
Nanograms	Nanograms Should not be abbreviated	↓		

There are other ways of expressing measurements for drugs and these will be discussed in more detail in relation to calculations as we move through the book (see Box 2).

Box 2   Measurement types and explanations

Measurement	Explanation
Grams, milligrams, micrograms and nanograms	Measures of a drug's weight, for example 1 gram paracetamol
Weight/volume	Some drugs are expressed according to the amount of weight of drug that has been dissolved in a certain amount of volume. For example, an elixir may contain 100mg/5ml (see Chapter 2)
Standardised International Units	These refer to a measurement of activity or effect of the drug. Each one unit of the drug has a specific biological effect, which is agreed internationally and is thus standardised. This varies for each drug. Quantities of the drug are then expressed as multiples of this standard
	The quantity of the drug has been standardised into 'units' of measurements, known as international units (IU), for example 25 000 units heparin (see Chapter 2 on units)
Percentages	Percentage refers to an amount of the drug standardised out of a hundred. For example, 5% glucose infusion refers to 5g out of every 100ml
Moles and millimoles (mmol/L)	Chemicals used as drugs, such as potassium, are expressed according to the number of atoms (smallest part of the chemical) that a solution contains. As atoms are very tiny, a measurement is often given for a specific number of atoms known as a 'mole'. There are also smaller measurements of the 'mole'. The most commonly seen in practice is the millimole (1 mole = 1000 millimoles). For example, an infusion may contain 40 millimoles of potassium in 1 litre. This is written as 40mmol/L
Ratios	Measurements can be expressed as a relationship between two parts. In drugs this is usually the relationship between the weight of a drug and the volume it is dissolved in. The most common ratio used in practice is adrenaline, which is often used in strengths 1:1000 or 1:100. This means that there is 1g of adrenaline to 1000ml (1:1000) or 1g adrenaline to 100ml (1:100) (see later in Chapter 1)

Weight

Most of us are familiar with kilograms (kg) and grams (g) as we use these measurements in everyday life, for example using 100g butter in a cake or buying a 2kg bag of sugar. (Although some of us are still more familiar with the old imperial system of pounds (lbs) and ounces (oz), we are at least aware and use the metric system on a daily basis.)

Kilograms and grams are useful measures for food where you need a relatively large amount. However, for drugs, where only a small amount may be needed to have a therapeutic effect, different weight measurements are required. This is where the other measurements of milligrams, micrograms and nanograms are useful (see Box 1).

> ## ✳ Clinical Context
>
> Only a tiny amount of digoxin is needed to have a therapeutic effect on a patient. If you only used the measurement of kilograms to express this weight of digoxin, you would have a prescription for 0.000000125kg! Obviously having such a number written on a medicine chart and on tablet bottles is cumbersome and likely to cause errors, with the risk of someone missing out one of the zeros. So in order to make it easier and safer to measure weight dosages for drugs, different, smaller units of measurements are required.

The order of size for the units of measurement and their common abbreviations can be seen in Box 1. In clinical practice, grams, milligrams and micrograms are the most common units used. When working in clinical areas where patients are clinically unstable, such as intensive care or theatres, or if working with young children and babies in paediatrics, much smaller amounts of drugs are required. In these areas the unit of measurement nanograms would also be used.

Drug dosages tend to be fairly stable in nursing, particularly in adult nursing, so that you begin to recognise the common dosages prescribed for certain drugs and the usual unit of measurement used. For example, I'm sure you have all seen paracetamol prescribed for adults as 1 gram, or amoxicillin for adults in milligrams.

Being able to recognise common drug dosages and their usual measurements will help you to form a picture in your head of what 1 gram looks like or 250 milligrams, for example. This will help when you are converting between different units of measurement (which I will explain shortly) and will also help you to check that any calculations you solve make sense for that particular drug.

Warning!

As nurses, we should always be familiar with the typical dosages for each drug before we administer these to ensure that there are no errors in either the prescription or our administration. Obviously it would be impossible to learn all the dosages for every single drug, which is why you should always have access to a drug formulary such as the *British National Formulary* (BNF) and use this to check before administering.

Formulations

Box 3   Common formulations for drugs

Formulation	Description
Tablets	Drug is mixed with a base to bind drug into a tablet form and then often coated with coloured material or sugar. Binding substance can be used to delay release of drug in stomach or intestine, for example slow release tablets
Capsules	Capsule containing the drug is made out of gelatine or a similar substance. Drug is released in the stomach or intestine as capsule is digested. Capsule substance can be used to delay the release of the drug
Elixir	Drug is dissolved in a liquid which usually contains alcohol and sweeteners
Mixtures	Liquids that contain several ingredients dissolved or diffused throughout water or another solvent
Emulsion	Two liquids where one is dispersed within the other
Linctus	A liquid that contains a syrupy substance to relieve coughs, for example codeine linctus
Ampoules or vials	A drug that has been dissolved in a liquid, usually water. If the drug is unstable in a liquid, it may be contained in the ampoule or vial as a powder form and require reconstituting prior to use, for example antibiotics

Drugs are manufactured in different formulations, for example tablets, elixirs and ampoules (see Box 3 for different formulations). For each formulation, the dose of drug contained is most commonly expressed in the weight that each amount of formulation contains of the drug. For example, for tablets and capsules the dosage in weight is given for each tablet, while for elixirs and ampoules it is the weight of drug that each set volume of the liquid contains, as illustrated below (Figure 1).

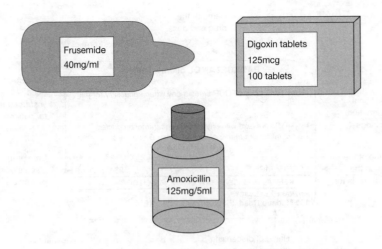

Figure 1 Medications and the dosages expressed as weight/volume
or weight for elixir, ampoules and tablets

> **Warning!**
> It is important that you check the medicine dosage carefully and under-
> stand what this means before beginning to calculate or administer it.

Labelling of Medications

Medicine that is kept as stock in a hospital ward is labelled by the drug
manufacturers and contains information about the name of medicine, the
dosage, expiry date and the number of tablets in the container/volume in
the container or ampoules in the box. This information needs to be checked
before you administer any medication (see Figure 2).

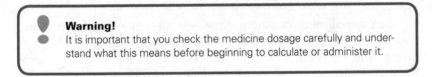

Name
of drug

Drug
manufacturer's
details here

Dose
of drug

Number
of tablets

Figure 2 Illustration of a medicine packet and labelling

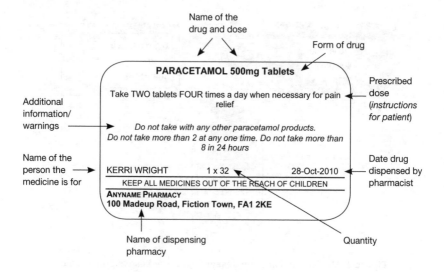

Figure 3 Medicine labelled for an individual person

When a medication has been dispensed for a specific person, it will have an additional administration label which has been added by the pharmacist. This can be a community pharmacist for people at home or a hospital pharmacist for people in a hospital or hospice (see Figure 3). This medicine must **only** be given to the person named on the label. The expiry date for this medicine will be on the side as before (see also Figure 4). A batch number refers to a group or batch of drugs that were produced at the same time by the manufacturers. This is useful if there is ever a problem with a drug as the manufacturers can track all drugs made at the same time (Figure 4).

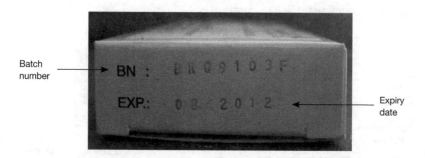

Figure 4 A side view of a medicine box showing the expiry date and batch number

Warning!
It is vital that you concentrate when you are calculating drug dosages and administering medication. You need to ensure that you create an environment that is as free as possible from distractions and allows you to concentrate. Ideally, complex dosage calculations should be undertaken in a room away from distractions, for example in a quiet room in a patient's house or a treatment room.

When you have medicine that is for an individual person, the dose prescribed and the amount of this medicine to be administered will have already been worked out by the pharmacist and put on the label. When you are using stock medicine, however, you need to calculate the amount to administer using the prescribed dosage. Generally, the prescribed dosage is written on a medicine administration chart (see Figure 5).

Sunnydene and Reynold NHS Trust

Name: Jarvis Maryland   **Hospital Number:** 01112348

Weight: 65kg   **Height:** 196cm

REGULAR PRESCRIPTIONS

Year 2011		Date & Month 1st February		Date Time												
Drug Phenytoin				07.00												
				09.00												
Dose 300mg	Route Po	Start date 1/2/11	Valid period 14 days	12.00												
				14.00												
Signature R Dickinson		Dispensed 1/2/11		18.00												
				22.00												

Figure 5 An example of a medicine administration chart

Looking at the medicine chart above, what dose of phenytoin does Jarvis require? Hopefully you can all read the information from the medicine chart that states that Jarvis has been prescribed 300mg phenytoin to be administered orally. As the nurse caring for Jarvis, you need to ensure that he receives this dose of phenytoin at the time prescribed.

On a ward, drugs are generally stocked in a drug trolley or in a patient's locked cupboard by their bed. Nurses take the required medicine from this stock. If the phenytoin tablets in stock each contain 100 milligrams of phenytoin, you would need to calculate how many tablets to give to Jarvis so that he received the required dose. I know this sounds obvious and you may be thinking that of course you would give three 100 milligram tablets to Jarvis because three lots of 100 milligrams would give 300 milligrams. If you have leapt to this solution then well done. Don't skip on to another section though, thinking that you know this and it's too easy. It is really important that you start to understand how you worked out the answer. This will help you in three ways to:

1.   Be safe and confident in the knowledge that your solution is correct
2.   Develop secure problem-solving skills for when you are faced with really tricky calculations
3.   Be able to explain to someone else why your answer is correct and support them with *their* calculations if necessary

It is important that you are secure in these fundamental steps of calculating so that you can build on these, knowing that your foundations are strong.

Warning!
It is important that you learn the different routes by which medications can be administered and also the abbreviations that are used on medicine administration charts. The route will give you information about the dose and whether it is likely to be correct and can also be useful in helping you to understand what it is you are trying to calculate, for example number of tablets to give for the patient to swallow or number of millilitres to inject (see Box 4).

With the example in Figure 5 you had to give a 300 milligram dose to Jarvis and you had tablets available which each contained 100 milligrams. Most people do one of two things when faced with a calculation like this:

1.   Either they 'see' immediately that 300 divided by 100 would be 3 so Jarvis would require 3 tablets.
2.   Or they 'see' that 100 milligrams add 100 milligrams add another 100 milligrams would give 300 milligrams, which is the required dosage so would be 3 tablets.

Box 4 Summary of the common routes, abbreviations and usual dose for this route

Route	Abbreviation	Forms	Usual dose
Orally	PO or O	Tablets, capsules, suspensions	1–5 tablets or between 1–50ml if suspension
Via PEG or NG tube PEG = percutaneous endoscopic gastrostomy tube NG = naso gastro tube	Via PEG or NG	Suspensions, elixirs	In liquid form so usually millilitres. Volume depends on dosage calculated for that medicine; usually more than 5ml. Medicine requires flushing with water to ensure it reaches the stomach and prevents tube blocking
Intramuscular injections	IM	Ampoules or vials* (may require reconstituting)	In liquid form so usually millilitres. Amount varies according to muscle site of injection and age of child but generally no more than 5ml
Intravenous	IV	Infusion bags, ampoules or vials* (may require reconstituting)	In liquid form and varies according to medication and how this needs to be administered, for example added to an infusion bag or as an injection
Subcutaneous	S/C or SC	Ampoules or vials* (may require reconstituting)	In liquid form so usually millilitres. Amount varies according to site for injection and age of child but generally no more than 2ml

* The terms ampoule or vial are often used interchangeably and refer to a small glass or plastic bottle that contains medicine in either a liquid or solid form (powder). I will be using both terms throughout this book.

The first method can be simplified and put into a formula that can be used each time this type of calculation is required. This formula is dividing the dosage of drug that the patient requires by the dosage contained in each tablet available. Most nurses shorten this formula to 'what you want divided by what you have'.

The second method is a repeated addition method and is often supported by the actions of the nurse during the physical act of administering the drug. For the above example, I would put each 100 milligram tablet into the dispensing pot and add up the total dosage contained until the prescribed dosage is reached. This method also allows the solution to be checked by actively counting the number of tablets as they are put into the pot: 1 tablet (= 100 milligrams), 2 tablets (= 200 milligrams), 3 tablets (= 300 milligrams). To check you have followed this, I am going to work through another example.

Example

You pick up a medicine chart for Mrs Davis who requires 30 milligrams prednisolone. You look in the drug trolley and the stock tablets available are 5 milligram tablets.

Formula method

$$\frac{\text{what you want}}{\text{what you have}} = \text{number of tablets}$$

$$\frac{30 \text{ milligrams}}{5 \text{ milligrams}}$$

$$= 6 \text{ tablets}$$

Repeated addition method

5 milligrams	1 tablet
10 milligrams	2 tablets
15 milligrams	3 tablets
20 milligrams	4 tablets
25 milligrams	5 tablets
30 milligrams	6 tablets

Of course there is nothing stopping you from using a combination of the two methods. For example, you might prefer the formula method, but then check your solution by repeatedly adding up the dosage weight contained in each tablet to check that it totals the required prescribed amount.

Before we move on, I need to take a slight detour. I know you are probably desperate to get on with it, but it is a vital and necessary detour at this stage.

● Checking

Often when students or nurses are solving drug calculations and especially when these are being practised from books or in a classroom setting, there is a tendency to rush to get to the answer and to check to see whether this is right. No problem here you may be thinking and yes, that is true, it is not a problem when you are in a classroom setting or sat at home. After all if you got the calculation wrong, all that happens is you have a look to see why, kick yourself for making such a silly mistake, correct it and move on. This is not the case in clinical practice. The answer that you reach is going to determine the dosage that you administer and if wrong ... well, I don't need to tell you what the implications could be. So, even if you are doing drug calculations at home or in a classroom it is vital that you get into the habit of checking your answer **as if** you were in clinical practice. It is precisely because we know that the dosage could cause harm to a patient if wrong that we do check and re-check in clinical practice (or at least we should do).

We need to get into the habit, in the classroom and at home, of thinking as if we were in practice and carry over these skills to the clinical setting. This means that when you arrive at your solution this is not the end point of your calculation at all. You need to carefully check this solution and your working out to ensure that you don't just **think** it is the right answer, but you **know** that it is right. Box 5 gives several ways for you to check that your answer is definitely correct. Please take the time to read this and practise these checking techniques. You can even photocopy this and pin it to your wall!

Box 5   Checking your solution to drug calculations

Checking
There are different ways that you can check that you have calculated the correct dosage. Some of the methods you would do naturally in a clinical setting and some you will need to train yourself to do. Some of the natural checks that you would do are not possible in a classroom, so in order to activate some of these natural checks you will need to imagine that you are in your clinical area and visualise actually preparing that dosage to administer.

Making sense
- The first obvious check is to look at your solution in the context of your understanding of the question and ask whether it fits as a solution here. So, does it make sense to administer that number of tablets or that volume of elixir considering what you are trying to work out?

For example, if you needed to give 10mg of a drug, the ampoules available are 50mg/1ml and you have worked out that you need to administer 5ml. Does this make sense? If 1ml contains 50mg then you need less than 1ml for 10mg so 5ml cannot be correct. This should stimulate you to relook at the question and see where you have gone wrong or try a different method for solving it.

● Estimate the answer or a range that you are expecting your answer to be within. The ideal situation would be for you to work out estimates for your solutions first, before you even start to solve the problem. However, you can also do them as you go along to check that you are on the right lines and also at the end to double-check your solutions.

For example, if you needed to administer 80mg and the ampoules were 100mg/2ml you can work out a range for this solution of between 1–2ml by using the halving method. The diagram below illustrates how to estimate the amount of solution to administer (and see, Chapter 2 for explanation of halving methods).

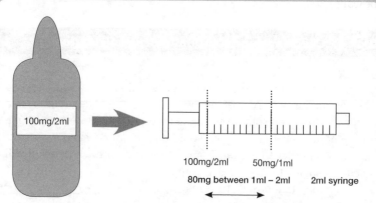

100mg/2ml   50mg/1ml
80mg between 1ml – 2ml   2ml syringe

Diagram illustrating how to estimate the amount of solution to administer

✔ **Tips for Learning**

Use the halving or doubling method to give you a rough estimate of what your answer should be (see Chapter 2, pages 45 and 48).

Practice experience

- You also need to look at your answer and think whether it makes sense in relation to clinical practice and your clinical experience. So have you ever administered 40 tablets to a patient? Have you ever had to draw up 5.3ml of a drug from ampoules before? Have you ever given 0.1ml of a suspension before? If you haven't done these things, this is not to say that you are wrong as there is a first time for everything, but it should ring a warning bell.

  The unfamiliarity of a drug dosage should trigger alarm bells, and make you stop and think about your calculation and whether it can be right. If, once you have checked and are convinced your calculation is correct, but it is still an unusual amount of the drug to give, then you need to check with someone else as it could be an error in the prescription. Even when you are in a classroom setting you should not think that just because you are not in clinical practice then any solution could be right. You should still keep the alarm bells active and use them as a warning for you.

- Use your clinical knowledge about specific drugs. So is this approximately the right volume that we give for this particular drug in your experience? As nurses, we need to be familiar with the drug dosages for any drugs that we administer and develop from experience what the expected amounts should be when administering drugs expressed as a weight and volume.

  When solutions for particular drugs fall outside our expected ranges, then alarm bells should again be triggered and prompt you to examine your solution again more carefully. Once again, if in doubt, you shouldn't be administering the drug and should be asking for someone else to check your calculation and the prescription written.

  To give an example using tablets, if you calculated that you needed to administer 4 paracetamol tablets you would immediately have an alarm bell ringing because you know that for adults the usual dosage is 2 tablets, so the calculated dosage of 4 immediately activates your warning system that something isn't quite right. Sometimes we don't always know what it is that isn't quite right, just that it doesn't seem right. That feeling of unease should be enough to trigger careful examination of your calculation and the prescription.

● Check backwards to ensure that you have got the right dosage to administer. For example, if you have worked out that you need to administer 3 tablets, then count up this dosage to ensure it equals the prescribed dosage. This is a common check to do, but can be lost if you are in a classroom or at home. In these instances you will need to imagine that you are preparing the dosage in your head and visualise counting the tablets.

Checking calculations

● Always go back over any calculations to check for understanding and any errors. To do this we can just work through our calculations again and check that we have done these correctly or we can work backwards and do the calculations a slightly different way. For example, if I had calculated that 125 divided by 5 is 25, then I could check this by multiplying 25 by 5 and ensuring I reached the same answer of 125.

Doing the calculation another way

● Check your solution to a calculation using another method. I have heard some nurses say that they will use a calculator to double-check that their solution is correct. However, in contrast, I have seen other nurses use a doubling and halving method to check the solution they reached using a calculator. Sometimes when you find the question difficult to understand and cannot obviously see the answer, using a calculator and the formula method can help to actually make sense of the question.

For example, if I had to administer 125mg of a drug and the elixir available was 50mg/5ml, I could use the formula method to give the solution to administer 12.5ml. Using this answer I could then work backwards to help me make sense of the answer and ensure it is correct. So here I may think 50mg/5ml, 100mg/10ml and 25mg/2.5ml so that would be 12.5ml.

There are quite a few different checks that you can and should be doing once your reach your solution. You must get into the habit of doing some of these each time you reach your solution or as you are working towards your solution. The most vital of these checks relies on your having a clear understanding of what that question is asking you to do. If you haven't got this understanding then you won't be able to look at your solution and see whether it actually makes sense. Many of these checking systems also rely on clinical experience so you must make sure that you practise these questions in a clinical situation as much as you can.

✔ Tips for Learning

It may not have escaped your notice that in order to solve problems such as this you need some mathematical knowledge. Thankfully, most drug dosages in clinical practice are nice easy numbers (particularly in adult nursing) so you can probably get away with working out 6 lots of 5 milligrams by adding up each 5 milligram and using your fingers to keep count of how many you have added. However, it would probably help you if you could recognise that $5 \times 6 = 30$ and therefore 6 tablets are required. The common dosages and multiples to learn are:

	×2	×3	×4	×5	×6	×7	×8	×9	×10	×20
5	10	15	20	25	30	35	40	45	50	100
10	20	30	40	50	60	70	80	90	100	200
15	30	45	60	75	90				150	300
20	40	60	80	100	120	140	160	180	200	400
25	50	75	100	125	150	175	200		250	500
50	100	150	200	250					500	1000
100	200	300	400	500	600	700	800	900	1000	2000
125	250	375	500	625			1000			
250	500	750	1000				2000			
500	1000	1500	2000							
1000	2000	3000	4000	5000	6000	7000	8000	9000	10 000	

For example, with the repeated addition method and an available tablet dose of 5mg then you would need to know your five times table!

For the formula method, if you have your calculator, then you need to understand that:

$$\frac{30 \text{ milligrams}}{5 \text{ milligrams}}$$

Mathematically, this actually means 30 milligrams divided by 5 milligrams or how many 5 milligrams there are in 30 milligrams. On your calculator you would therefore key in:

$\boxed{3}\;\boxed{0}\;\boxed{\div}\;\boxed{5}\;\boxed{=}$

If you did not have a calculator, then you would have to know that $30 \div 5 = 6$ (or work it out using repeated addition).

To check that you are really secure in these two methods I will give you some more calculations from practice. The answers and the working for both methods are available in the answers section.

EXERCISE 1

1. The medicine administration chart states that Joy requires 1000 milligrams of amoxicillin. The stock tablets available each contain 250 milligrams of amoxicillin. How many tablets do you need to administer to Joy?
2. Sita requires 250 micrograms of digoxin. The tablets available each contain 62.5 micrograms. How many tablets would you administer to Sita?

(Answers: page 215)

✔ **Tips for Learning**

When buying a calculator for nursing, please consider the following guidance:

- You only need the four arithmetic functions of addition, subtraction, multiplication and division. Avoid using calculators that have more complex functions unless you are confident in using these
- Use an actual calculator rather than a calculator function on a mobile phone or computer
- Ensure that the calculator keys are the right size for your fingers. You need to be able to accurately key in the numbers and function

you want. Bigger keys are better and reduce the risk of pressing
the wrong key by mistake
- Make sure that the screen is clear enough for you to read the
numbers easily, bearing in mind that you may be using this when
you are tired or the light is poor
- Try to use your own calculator consistently so you become used to
how it works and the feel of the keys
- Always carry your calculator with you on duty if you are regularly
calculating drug dosages and prefer to use a calculator for this

● Converting

There are times in clinical practice when you need to express the unit of
measurement used for a drug in another unit of measurement. For example,
you may want to express 1 gram of paracetamol in milligrams or 0.1 milligram of aminophylline in micrograms. The most common time when you
need to do this conversion is when the prescribed drug has been expressed
in a different unit of measurement to the stock drug available. For example,
the prescription may stipulate 0.25 milligrams of digoxin, but the stock
tablets available on the ward or in someone's home are 62.5 microgram
tablets. One dosage (in this case the prescription) is expressing the weight
in milligrams and the other (tablets) is expressing the weight in micrograms.
You cannot follow the same procedure as before to work out how many
tablets you need to administer to give this dosage because the unit of measurement for each dosage is different. This is like trying to compare euros
with dollars or kilograms with stones. The only way to compare the two
dosages in order to calculate how many tablets to give is to convert both
dosages into the *same* unit of measurement.

To convert between different units of measurement you need to know
the relationship between them. This is the same as when you are on holiday
and you want to understand how much money those classy jeans cost: you
would convert the price given in dollars into sterling, that is, pounds. So
you would work out that if $1 = £2 then the $25 jeans would cost £50 and
are not quite the bargain you thought!

Thankfully, for converting between weights in clinical practice the
'conversion rate' stays stable (unlike currency rates) and is the same
conversion amount between all the units of weight. So you only need to
remember one number. That magic number is 1000.

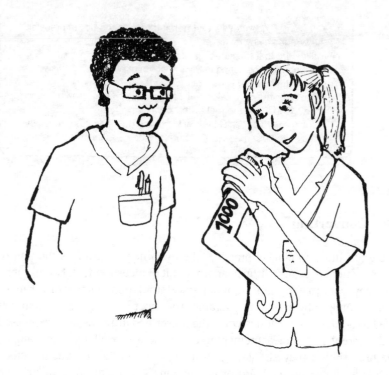

Using this relationship we know that:

1 kilogram = 1000 grams
1 gram = 1000 milligrams
1 milligram = 1000 micrograms
1 microgram = 1000 nanograms (see Box 6)

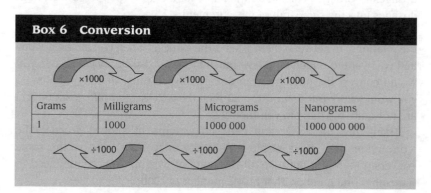

Box 6   Conversion

Grams	Milligrams	Micrograms	Nanograms
1	1000	1000 000	1000 000 000

×1000   ×1000   ×1000

÷1000   ÷1000   ÷1000

Using this relationship, how many milligrams would be the same weight as 0.5 grams? Look back at Box 6 if you are not sure.

Just remember the 1000 relationship and you'll be halfway there. When converting between different weights, it will help you considerably if you can visualise in some way what it is you are doing. To be able to visualise this, it is helpful to be secure in your knowledge of the different units of weight and the size order of each of these. For example, if you can picture and understand that micrograms are 1000 times smaller than milligrams, you will be able to 'see' that you will need a thousand micrograms to make up the same weight as 1 milligram. This is the same as saying that you need 1000 mice to equal the same weight as 1 elephant! Have a look at Figure 6 below to help you imagine this.

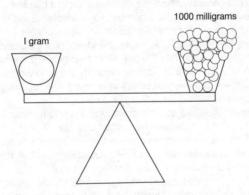

Figure 6 Illustrating the relationship between grams and milligrams

Remember that 1000 milligrams is the same weight as 1 gram so you need a thousand times more milligrams to equal the equivalent weight of grams. To work out how many milligrams is the same weight as 0.5 grams, therefore, you could do one of three things:

1. You could multiply 0.5 grams by 1000 (if you are unsure about multiplying and dividing by 1000 please go to Chapter 4 where this is explained in detail).

2. You could use the knowledge that 1 gram is the same weight as 1000 milligrams, so 0.5 is one half of 1 gram. Therefore the equivalent weight would be one half of 1000 milligrams.

3. Finally, you could use your practice knowledge of different drug dosages and know that one paracetamol tablet contains 500 milligrams, which is a half of 1 gram.

Hopefully you have worked out that the answer is 500 milligrams.

Many nurses in practice are able to 'see' the equivalent weights in different units of measurement through experience and through repetition of similar conversions. As you practise these conversions, they will become more familiar and easier to you. The best way of practising is always in clinical practice where you can make sense of the whole calculation required in relation to the clinical care for specific patients and actually have the tablets and medicine charts in front of you. Before we move on to more clinical examples it would be an idea to explain and practise conversions a bit more.

Warning!

We do not generally show the decimal point in a number unless the number is a part of a whole number, for example 1.2, although the decimal point is still there. So I could write the number 1 as 1.000 showing that it is 1 unit, no tenths, hundredths of thousandths and so on (this is explained more in Chapter 4). In healthcare, there have been a number or errors in drug administration through the written numbers being unclear and misread or misunderstood. The following rules have been devised to help prevent these errors:

- Never include a decimal point after a whole number, for example 2.0. This must always be written clearly as 2
- A zero or number should always come before a decimal point, for example 3.6 or 0.6, we should not be writing .7 as the decimal can easily be missed and the number read as 7
- When writing large numbers commas should not be used. These can be misread as decimal points. In some countries, commas are used as decimal points, which can lead to confusion. It is clearer to use a space, for example 5000 000
- If there is any doubt that the dose maybe misread, then the number can be written in both numerical figures and words in the same way as when writing on a cheque. This system is used when controlled drugs are being prescribed, for example 240mg morphine sulphate, two hundred and forty milligrams morphine sulphate

✔ Tips for Learning

Some written drug calculation tests may have questions that ask you to convert from grams to micrograms or micrograms to grams. If this is the case, then do your conversion in stages. First convert the grams to milligrams and then the milligrams to micrograms. This will help you to be more systematic and reduce errors.

In practice, most of the conversions required will be between grams and milligrams; milligrams and micrograms; or micrograms and nanograms. Very rarely, if ever, would you need to convert between grams and micrograms or grams and nanograms! In addition in clinical practice, you would not be required to convert dosage after dosage into different units of measurement, first going from grams to milligrams and then micrograms to milligrams as is often required in written drug calculation tests. This can become quite confusing. To try to avoid this, we will do each conversion in turn and practise these and then at the end of the chapter you can practise these all mixed up as you would find in a written test. If you are not feeling confident about these conversions, then use Box 6 to help you or think about common drug dosages you know in practice.

Warning!
You must clearly state the unit of measurement in your answer. The answer of 200 would not be correct as this does not state whether this is units, grams or sack loads of the drug!

EXERCISE 2

Grams to milligrams
Convert the following gram weights into the equivalent milligram weights:
1.   0.6 grams
2.   1.2 grams
3.   0.25 grams

Milligrams to grams
Convert the following milligram weights into equivalent gram weights:
1.   1800 milligrams
2.   800 milligrams
3.   2000 milligrams

Milligrams to micrograms
Convert the following milligram weights into equivalent microgram weights:
1.   0.3 milligrams
2.   0.125 milligrams
3.   0.01 milligrams

Micrograms to milligrams
Convert the following microgram weights into equivalent milligram weights:
1.   100 micrograms
2.   500 micrograms
3.   2500 micrograms

(Answers: page 215)

✔ **Tips for Learning**

When completing written tests read the questions carefully and do not assume that the questions will represent reality and accidentally 'read' milligrams instead of micrograms as this is what you are expecting.

Having become more confident with conversions, we will now consider a conversion within a calculation in clinical practice. For example, Ali has been prescribed 1.8 grams benzylpenicillin and the ampoules available each contain 600mg. There are several stages to this calculation:

1. You need to be clear that you understand what it is you are trying to work out. In this problem it is how many ampoules or part of the ampoules you need to administer in order for Ali to receive the required prescription dose of 1.8 grams.
2. You should recognise that the units of measurement being used for the dosages are different so you will need to convert one of the dosages. So you now need to work out how many milligrams would be the same weight as 1.8 grams.

Using your understanding of the different units of weight, you know that:

- Milligrams are lighter than grams
- 1000 milligrams are required to make up the equivalent weight of 1 gram
- To convert from grams to milligrams therefore, you need a thousand times more milligrams. So you would need to multiply 1.8 grams by 1000 (see Box 6 to help you if you are unsure)

Once you have done this multiplication, you should arrive at the answer that 1.8 grams in equivalent milligram weight is 1800 milligrams.

3. You now need to go back to the question that you were asked again. Your patient requires 1800 milligrams of benzylpenicillin and the ampoules available each contain 600 milligrams of benzylpenicillin. Remember, you are working out how many ampoules you need to administer to give the 1800 milligram prescribed dosage. Hopefully you can now recognise that the problem is the same as previous questions on working out how

many tablets to give. So you should now be able to work out how many ampoules to give using one of the methods I showed you. If you can't remember or didn't recognise this problem, don't worry. It will come in time, providing that you continue practising!

To work out this problem you can use either of the two methods I have already shown you:

Formula

$$\frac{1800 \text{ milligrams}}{600 \text{ milligrams}}$$

= 3 ampoules

Repeated addition

600 milligrams	1 ampoule
1200 milligrams	2 ampoules
1800 milligrams	3 ampoules

We can summarise the steps that you followed to solve this problem (see Box 7).

As you become more experienced, you won't think through each step like this but will probably 'jump' straight to the answer of 3 ampoules. I am sure that you have seen nurses do this in practice and have been left in admiration wondering how they worked it out so quickly! As you are developing this expertise, though, it is useful to go keep going through these steps systematically to ensure you understand exactly what it is you are doing and why.

Being systematic is also really important when you start to solve more complex calculations and time spent developing this approach now will help you in the future. In addition, even when you become more of an expert and are able to 'jump' straight to the answers, it is still essential that you are able to think back to the steps that you have taken automatically and without consciously thinking about them so that you can explain your solution to other nurses and also support learners as they develop calculation skills. Using the steps in Box 5 to guide your thinking, have a go at solving the clinical problems in Exercise 3.

After you have completed this exercise I will assume that you are more confident with units of measurements for weight and will therefore revert to only using their abbreviations rather than their full names as I have been doing so far. You can always check in Box 1 if you are ever unsure.

✔ Tips for Learning

You can either convert the prescription dosage from grams to milligrams or the ampoule dosage from milligrams to grams. Which one do you think would be easier? Generally the **rule is to convert to the same unit of measurement that the available drug is expressed in**. So, in this example, you would convert the prescription of 1.8 grams into milligram weight. Why do you think this rule makes the calculation easier? What would happen if we converted the 600 milligram ampoules into grams?

Example
You require 1.8 grams and have ampoules of 600 milligrams. To demonstrate, we will convert 600 milligrams into grams, so 600 ÷ 1000 = 0.6g. You now need to find out how many of these will make 1.8 grams. You can do this by adding up 0.6 until you reach 1.8 or dividing 1.8 by 0.6. You will get the same answer as before, but the decimal point can cause confusion and possible errors.

✔ Tips for Learning

If the size of the numbers is putting you off, you could imagine that it is 18 and 6 you are dealing with (reducing down by dividing both by 100). You can do this with either method, so you are dividing 18 by 6 and repeatedly adding sixes.

Box 7 Step by step guide – calculating number of tablets or ampoules to administer

1. Think about what you are actually trying to work out, for example how many tablets to administer, how much of an ampoule to administer and so on.
2. Check the units of measurement in prescribed dosage and available drug dosage are the same.
3. If the units of measurement are different, then convert the prescribed dosage units into the available drug units.
4. Go back to the question and recheck what you are trying to work out using the new measurements.

5. Work out how many tablets or ampoules to administer using the formula method or repeated addition.

6. Check that your answer makes sense in relation to the question and clinical practice, for example is it usual in practice to give this number of tablets? Is this the usual number of tablets to give for this drug? If you gave this number of tablets, what dosage would you be giving (add up the dosage for each tablet and check it is the same as the prescribed dosage).

✔ Tips for Learning

The words 'what you want' do not always feature in written drug calculation questions. The 'what you want' is basically the dosage that you want to give to someone because it is the dosage prescribed. So you will see different expressions such as 'you need to give', 'you are required to give', 'your patient has been prescribed' or 'the patient needs', for example. These all have the same meaning, which is the dosage that you are going to give to the patient, that is, what you want to administer.

EXERCISE 3

1. Your patient has been prescribed 0.25 milligrams digoxin. The tablets available each contain 62.5 micrograms. How many tablets would you administer?

2. Your patient has been prescribed 1.2 grams benzylpenicillin. The ampoules available each contain 600 milligrams. How many ampoules would you administer?

3. John requires 1 gram amoxicillin. The tablets available each contain 250 milligrams. How many tablets do you need to administer?

4. Your patient requires 0.1 grams of flucloxacillin. The elixir contains 100 milligrams in every 5 millilitres. How many millilitres would you administer?

5. Ola has been prescribed 0.3 milligrams hyoscine. The hyoscine ampoules each contain 600 micrograms. How many or how much of the ampoule would you administer?

(Answers: page 216)

● Units

There is another measurement used in clinical practice to express dosages which are known as Standardised International Units (SIU). In clinical practice you will see these dosages written as Units or abbreviated to 'U' or IU (International Units). For example, you may see a dose of 50U insulin or 25 000 units heparin. Units are weights of specific drugs which have been standardised according to their therapeutic activity level. This basically means that they are easier to use! The most common drugs you will probably come across that are expressed as standardised units are insulin and heparin.

Warning!

I must quickly give a word of warning about insulin. Insulin dosages, as I have mentioned, are standardised into units. The units are standardised so that 100 units are contained in 1ml. In the past nurses had to work out how many millilitres to draw up to administer a certain number of units of insulin using this principle. For example, if the dose was 23 units the nurse would have to calculate what proportion of 1ml to administer! (Who said the old ways are best!). Nowadays in clinical practice, we have insulin syringes that are calibrated to give the units along the side. So we only have to draw up the insulin to the required 23 units marked on the syringe.

There is a warning here, though, which is **ensure that you are using the right syringe when drawing up insulin**. Sadly, a community nurse gave a fatal dose of insulin to her patient by drawing up the units of insulin in a 1ml syringe and giving millilitres of insulin rather than the required unit dosage given on an insulin syringe (Stokes, 2009).

● Ratios

Ratios are another way of specifying the dosage of a drug. Ratios express a relationship between two amounts (see Chapter 4 for more information on ratios). In drug dosages, this is usually the weight of the drug in relation to the volume. The most common drug that is expressed as a ratio is adrenaline. Adrenaline is manufactured in several different strengths – 1:100, 1:1000 and 1:10 000 strength. The adrenaline is expressed here as a weight in relation to the volume that it has been dissolved in. This ratio in practice means:

1:1000 = 1g adrenaline for very 1000ml
1:100 = 1g adrenaline for every 100ml

Generally, any ratio in practice also has the weight volume dosage written on the drug as well. For adrenaline the weight/volume dosage would be:

1:10 000   100mcg/1ml
1:1000   1mg/1ml
1:100   10mg/1ml

To understand why these two ways of expressing the dosage are the same see Box 8.

Box 8   Explanation of dosages used for adrenaline

1:1000 means 1g in 1000ml. This could be written as a weight/volume dose as 1g/1000ml. If we convert the adrenaline dosage to milligrams this would be 1000mg/1000ml. We can now divide both sides by 1000 to get 1mg/1ml (remembering the rule of doing the same to each side).

For the 1:100 dosage:

1g in 100ml	
1000mg in 100ml	convert grams to milligrams
10mg in 1 ml	divide both sides by 100

For the 1:10 000 dosage:

1g in 10 000ml	
1000mg in 10 000ml	convert grams to milligrams
0.1mg in 1ml	divide both sides by 1000
100mcg in 1ml	converting milligrams to micrograms

In practice, you would rarely need to calculate dosages using ratios alone and it is enough to appreciate the different strengths that ratios represent. However, ratio calculations can sometimes be used in written drug calculation assessments and so it is worth ensuring that you understand these. Try these three questions which could appear in a written test:

EXERCISE 4

1. How many milligrams of 1:1000 adrenaline are contained in 0.5ml?
2. You administer 2ml 1:100 adrenaline. How many milligrams of adrenaline have you administered?
3. You need to administer 200mcg adrenaline. How many millilitres of 1:10 000 adrenaline would you need to give?

(Answers: page 217)

● Dosage per Weight

In order to have the precise therapeutic effect, some medication is prescribed according to the patient's individual body weight. The same dosage of medication would have a different effect on a larger person compared with a smaller person. This is especially important where someone's clinical condition is unstable and medication needs to be given more precisely and also in children where individual weights vary greatly.

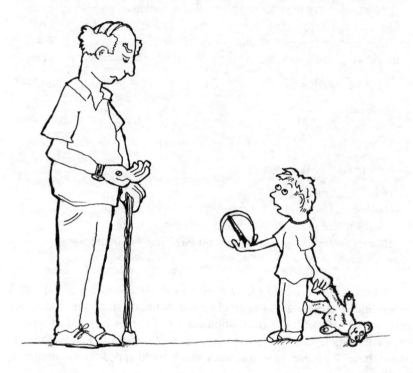

When a medication has been prescribed according to body weight it is usually prescribed as a specific weight of medication for every kilogram weight of the individual. So, for example, the prescription could be 2mg/kg. This means that for every kilogram the person weighs they need 2mg. So if the individual weighed 2 kilograms you would give 2mg for the first kilogram and then 2mg for the second kilogram weight. The dosage required for this person would thus be 2 lots of 2mg, which would be 4mg.

> ✳ **Clinical Context**
>
> Some drugs, such as chemotherapy, are prescribed according to the body surface area (BSA) of the patient, for example $2mg/m^2$ (this is more common in children). Once you have calculated the surface area, then the calculation proceeds in the same way as a dosage per weight calculation. The calculation for the BSA relies on a formula and there are several available to use. It is recommended that you refer to your clinical area for the advised BSA formula to use.

If your patient weighed 10kg and you needed to give 2mg/kg how many milligrams would this person require?

Remember that for every kilogram weight of the patient you need to give 2mg, so here you would need to give ten lots of 2mg. This would be 20mg. Do you understand what you are doing mathematically to work out the dosage? How would you explain the way to work out weight dosages to someone who didn't know? Have a look at the following example to see if you are correct.

Example

You are required to administer a certain dosage for every kilogram weight of the individual. So for every kilogram that the person weighs you administer that dosage. If the prescription was 10mcg/kg and the person weighed 5kg, you would need to administer:

10mcg (1kg) and 10mcg (1kg) and 10mcg (1kg) and 10mcg (1kg) and 10mcg (1kg) = 50mcg/5kg

This is 5 lots of 10mcg, which is the same as saying 10mcg multiplied by 5 or mathematically 5×10.

The formula for working out the weight/dosage is: weight of person (kg) × dosage per kg

Using this formula what is the total dosage required for a patient who has been prescribed 5mg/kg and who weighs 25kg?

weight of person (kg) = 25
dosage per kg = 5mg
So, $25 \times 5mg$
= 125mg to administer

> ✔ **Tips for Learning**
>
> Always keep the units of measurement if writing down the calculation as above. If using a calculator, make sure that you go back to the question to check what unit of measurement your answer is in.

> ? **Maths Explained**
>
> You will find that knowledge of long multiplication could be helpful for you here. Have a look at Chapter 4 where this is explained.

Warning!
To ensure that your patient is receiving the correct dose of the medication with dose/weight prescriptions, it is important that the weight of the patient you are using in the calculation is accurate. This means that you will need to consider how and how often you ascertain the weight of your patient in order to use this figure in your calculations. For example, do you weigh your patient? When was your patient last weighed and is their weight likely to have changed since then? Also, consider the accuracy of relying on patients' or parents' recall of their own or their child's weight.

Once you have worked out the dosage of drug for that particular patient, you can then proceed with calculating how many tablets or ampoules to administer to the patient using the stock drug available. This means that for some problems in clinical practice there are actually several stages that you need to work out in order to solve the problem. These stages have been summarised in Box 9.

This is similar to the stages you work through in order to calculate the number of tablets or ampoules to administer when the units of measurement used for the two dosages are different, but with the additional stage of calculating the dosage the individual patient requires first. Again, once you become more familiar with these problems in clinical practice, you will be able to work through these stages in your head or jump some stages. However, as you are developing competence in calculation skills it is recommended that you follow each stage and become familiar with this sequencing and way of thinking first.

Box 9   Step by step guide – calculating number of tablets or ampoules to administer when prescribed as dose per weight

1. Make sure you understand the question and what exactly you are trying to work out. For example, the dosage for the individual patient and then how much of the available drug to give in order to administer this dosage.

2. Calculate the individual dose for the patient by multiplying their weight in kilograms by the dosage per kilogram.

3. Go back to the question and check that you are still clear about your understanding. For example, I know the actual dosage I now need to calculate how much of the available drug to administer.

4. Check that the prescribed dosage has the same unit of measurements as the available drug dosage.

5. If the units of measurement are different, then convert the prescribed dosage so it is expressed in the same unit of measurement as the available drug.

6. Go back to the question and check that you are still clear about your understanding. For example, I need to administer this dosage, I have this dosage available and they are both now in the same unit of measurement. I now need to work out how much of this drug would give the prescribed dosage.

7. Work out how much of the available drug to administer by using repeated addition or dividing the prescribed dosage by the available dosage.

8. Check your answer makes sense in relation to the questions and the dosages being prescribed and available, and your knowledge of clinical practice. For example, does it seem reasonable to administer this amount of a drug? Have I ever administered this amount before? Is this the usual amount of ampoules/tablets that I administer for this particular drug?

EXERCISE 5

1. Your patient has been prescribed 50mg/kg of amoxicillin. Your patient weighs 10kg. The amoxicillin ampoules available contain 250mg. How many of these ampoules do you need to administer to your patient in order to give the prescribed dosage?
2. Your patient has been prescribed 2mg/kg gentamicin. Your patient weighs 60kg. The available ampoules of gentamicin each contain 40mg/1ml. How many of these gentamicin ampoules would you administer to give the prescribed dosage?
3. Your patient has been prescribed 500mcg/kg of frusemide by slow intramuscular injection. Your patient weighs 10kg. The frusemide ampoules available are 10mg/ml. How many millilitres would you administer?

(Answers: page 218)

● **Divided Doses**

Some prescriptions do not specify what dosage the patient requires throughout the day, but will specify a total dosage over the 24-hour period and the number of doses required. For example, instead of the usual prescription of 50mg diclofenac sodium required at 9am, 2pm and 10pm, it may be prescribed as 150mg in three divided dosages per day. So the patient needs three equal doses of the drug throughout the day. With this example, how many milligrams would you administer for each dose?

In order to gain three equal doses I need to 'share' 150mg between three dosages. This means that I need to divide 150mg by 3 to work out that I would administer 50mg of the drug, at three separate times spread throughout the day. The doses obviously need to be spaced out equally throughout the day.

Most regular dosages are given during the day, usually between 6am and 10pm on a standard ward. So the three dosages of 50mg may be administered at 9am, 2pm and 10pm, although any times that are roughly equally spaced out throughout the day would be acceptable.

To summarise, if the total dosage for the day has been prescribed with the number of divided dosages required for the day, then to calculate this you divide the total dosage by the number of dosages required:

$$\frac{\text{total daily dosage}}{\text{number of dosages required}} = \text{dosage each time}$$

Try the following questions:

EXERCISE 6

1. Your patient has been prescribed 500mg in four divided dosages throughout the day. What dosage would you administer each time?
2. Your patient has been prescribed 1800mg in three divided dosages throughout the day. What dosage would you administer each time?
3. Your patient has been prescribed 1g in two divided dosages throughout the day. What dosage would you administer each time?

(Answers: page 219)

● Chapter Summary

This chapter has explained the different types of measurements that are used to express the dosages of drugs and how we convert between them. I have also explained how to calculate the number of tablets to administer to a patient and how to calculate divided doses and the dose when expressed as a dose per patient weight.

Now have a go at the assessment for this chapter.

Assessment 1

1. Your patient has been prescribed 500mg amoxicillin orally. The tablets available are 250mg tablets. How many tablets do you need to administer to your patient?

2. The doctor has prescribed 60mg/kg cefuroxine in three divided doses for a child who weighs 18kg. What dose does the child require for each administration?

3. You need to administer 2g flucloxcillin to your patient. The tablets available are 500mg tablets. How many tablets do you need to administer?

4. Using the information on the medicine chart below and the available digoxin tablets, calculate how many tablets you would administer to Mr Kumar.

Sunnydene and Reynold NHS Trust

Name: Fred Kumar   **Hospital Number:** 0789655

Weight: 76kg   **Height:** 178cm

REGULAR PRESCRIPTIONS

Year 2011		Date & Month 1st February		Date Time											
Drug Digoxin				07.00											
				09.00											
Dose 0.5mg	Route PO	Start date 1/2/11	Valid period 14 days	12.00											
				14.00											
Signature R Dickinson		Dispensed 1/2/11		18.00											
				22.00											
Additional comments															
Drug Gentamicin				07.00											
				09.00											
Dose 2mg/kg	Route IM	Start date 1/2/11	Valid period 2 days	12.00											
				14.00											
Signature R Dickinson		Dispensed 1/2/11		18.00											
				22.00											
Additional comments															

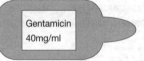

Digoxin tablets
125mcg   Flash drug manufacturer
100 tablets

Gentamicin
40mg/ml

5. Use the information from the medicine chart above to calculate the dose of gentamicin that Mr Kumar requires.

6. Your patient requires 30mg prednisolone. The tablets available are 5mg. How many tablets do you need to administer?

7. Your patient has been prescribed 1.2g benzylpenicillin. The vials contain 600mg. How many vials will you need to administer?

8. Your patient has been prescribed 3mg/kg daily of spironolactone in three divided doses. The patient weighs 50kg. The tablets available are 25mg. How many tablets does your patient require for each dose?

9. You need to give 300mg phenytoin to your patient orally. The tablets available are 100mg. How many do you need to administer?

10. You need to administer 50mg/kg daily chloramphenicol in four divided doses. Your patient weighs 40kg and the capsules available are 250mg. How many capsules would you need to administer for each dose?

(Answers: page 219)

References

Stokes, P. (2009) Pensioner 'unlawfully killed' by nurse's insulin overdose, *The Daily Telegraph* online at http://www.telegraph.co.uk/news/uknews/5061193/Pensioner-unlawfully-killed-by-nurses-insulin-over-dose.html (last accessed 1/7/10).

2 The Next Step! Medicines expressed as weight/volume strengths

66_Building on the foundations and tackling more complex calculations_**99**

This chapter explores:

▶ An outline of different methods to calculate medication doses for medicines expressed as a weight/volume strength

▶ Calculating medication dose from prescriptions based on patients' body weight for medicines expressed as weight/volume strength

▶ Calculations involving medications that require reconstituting

● Weight/Volume

So far we have mainly concentrated on some of the fundamental calculations that you will be required to solve in clinical practice focusing on drug dosages that are expressed in weights only. Now we are going to build on these skills by looking some more at drug dosages that are expressed as a weight and a volume. These calculations are slightly trickier, as you are dealing with weights and volumes together, but use similar strategies to those I've have shown you so far.

You will still need to convert between different units of measurement (see converting, page 19) and work out dosages per kilogram weight for individual patients, for example. And on top of this you will also have to manipulate dosages of drugs expressed in weight and volume.

Drug dosages are expressed as a weight and a volume when the drug formulation is an elixir, syrup or ampoule. Elixirs or syrups help swallowing or allow the medicine to be administered through a PEG tube (percutaneous endoscopic gastrostomy tube) and ampoules enable the drug to be injected (see Box 10).

Box 10   Syringes

Medications dosages that are in a liquid form are expressed in volume measurements usually millilitres (ml) or litres (L). Administration is by injection using various routes, orally or via a PEG tube. The method of measurement is usually a syringe. Syringes come in different volume sizes (see Figure 13) and in different types depending on the method of administration. Volumes can be measured using the scales on the side of each syringe.

Syringes can have needles already attached, for example insulin needles, or can be attached to different size needles. There are also oral syringes and measuring spoons, which are useful for measuring and administering elixirs, specifically in paediatric nursing.

The large volume syringes (10ml, 20ml and 50ml) are manufactured in two different types: as a normal syringe for attachment to needles and with a leur lock. A 'leur lock' is a syringe with a screw-like mechanism on the end, which twists and locks onto infusion lines (see Figure 7). These are useful for continuous infusions of medicine (see Chapter 3).

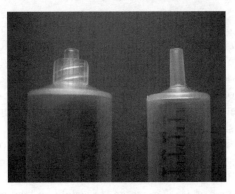

Figure 7 A normal syringe end and a syringe with a leur lock

✳ Clinical Context

Paediatric nurses tend to do a lot of calculations involving weight and volume as most children find it difficult to swallow tablets so elixirs are often prescribed. So if you are working in this area, it is especially important that you become confident with these calculations.

Elixirs and liquid ampoules are liquid, so the dosage of the drug needs to be expressed as the weight contained in a specific volume of liquid. To help understand what is happening with these dosages, it is helpful to get a basic idea of how ampoules and elixirs are constituted, that is, made. First, though, I will start with an example of a cup of tea to illustrate this.

Consider a cup of tea to which you add two teaspoons of sugar, as you are tired at the end of a long day. You stir in the sugar so it is all dissolved. Your cup of tea now contains two teaspoons of sugar. If you drank the whole cup of tea you would have 'eaten' two teaspoons of sugar. When elixirs and ampoules are made, the same thing happens to the drug as the sugar in your cup of tea.

Now consider Figure 8. In this illustration 10 grams of a drug have been added to 100ml water. The drug has been stirred until it has all dissolved. The solution that has been made now contains 10 grams of the drug dissolved in 100ml water. If you were to give the whole 100ml you would have administered 10g of the drug.

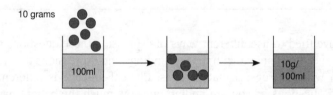

Figure 8 Demonstration of how a weight/volume dosage is 'manufactured'

The volume now contains the weight of the drug. Drug ampoules and elixirs will specify on the labels how much weight of the drug has been dissolved in how much liquid. Usually this information will be written as weight/volume for example 10g/100ml. This means 10 grams of the drug have been dissolved in 100ml as shown in Figure 8. So, if a morphine ampoule is labelled 30mg/1ml, this tells me that 30mg weight of morphine has been dissolved in 1ml. If I were to administer the whole ampoule, that is, 1ml, I would therefore be administering 30mg of morphine to my patient.

Warning!
Drugs are manufactured in different strengths. For example, morphine sulphate ampoules are available in strengths such as 10mg/1ml, 15mg/1ml, 20mg/1ml and 30mg/1ml, so it is vital that each ampoule label is checked carefully to ensure you know exactly what dose of the drug it contains.

Just to ensure that you are clear on the principle of weight and volume formulations before we move on, have a go at these questions (they are not trick questions!).

EXERCISE 7

1. The ampoule contains 40mg/ml. What weight of the drug have you given if you administer the whole ampoule?
2. The elixir contains 50mg/5ml. What volume would you give to administer 50mg?
3. The ampoule contains 20mg/2ml. You want to administer 20mg. How many millilitres would you administer?
4. Your patient has been prescribed 1mg of a drug. The ampoules available are 1mg/1ml. How many millilitres would you administer?
5. Your patient has been prescribed 10mg. The elixir strength is 10mg/5ml. What volume of elixir would you administer?

(Answers: page 219)

I have tried to use different ways of expressing these questions so you start to become familiar with the terminology and expressions that you will find in written drug calculation tests. Clinical practice is different from written questions as you are finding out how much the patient has been prescribed from a medicine chart and the strength of the elixir and ampoule from the label, but it is useful to develop both skills since you will often be tested using a written drug calculation test. Use the medicine chart and drug information below to complete the following exercise.

EXERCISE 8

Sunnydene and Reynold NHS Trust

Name: Millish Mackree   **Hospital Number:** 0045455

Weight: 63kg   **Height:** 162cm

REGULAR PRESCRIPTIONS

Year 2011	Date & month 1st February	Date Time							
Drug Metoclopramide hydrochloride		07.00							
		09.00							

Dose	Route	Start date	Valid period	12.00							
5mg	1M	1/2/11	14 days	14.00							
Signature		Dispensed		18.00							
R Dickinson		1/2/11		22.00							
Additional comments											
Drug				07.00							
Morphine sulphate				09.00							
Dose	Route	Start date	Valid period	12.00							
20mg	IM	1/2/11	2 days	14.00							
Signature		Dispensed		18.00							
R Dickinson		1/2/11		22.00							
Additional comments											

Medication available

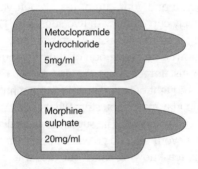

1. Calculate how many millilitres/ampoules of the available metoclopramide you would administer to Millish.
2. How many millilitres/ampoules of the available morphine sulphate would you administer to Millish?

(Answers: page 220)

You should have got the idea that the volume expressed on the ampoule or elixir bottle contains the stated weight of the drug. So if you administer all of that volume you will be administering the stated drug weight. This is nice and straightforward when the prescribed dosage for the patient is the same as the dosage per volume expressed on the stock drug ampoule or bottle.

When the prescribed dose is different, however, it means working out how much of the volume would contain the required dosage. For example, if your patient had been prescribed 5mg of a drug and the ampoule contains 20mg/2ml the dosage prescribed is different from the ampoule strength (see Figure 9).

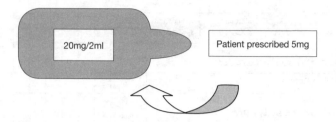

Figure 9 Patient requires only 5mg from the 20mg/2ml ampoule

Administering the whole ampoule volume of 2ml would administer 20mg. This is far too much, as we only need to give 5mg. So we need to work out what volume of this ampoule would contain the drug weight of 5mg. This can be slightly trickier.

Let's go back to you and your cup of tea. We left you sitting with your feet up hugging a lovely cup of tea with two sugars in. There you are sitting contentedly and are about to take a sip when suddenly you remember your diet! You are only allowed one teaspoon of sugar in your tea.

Grr! You want to just forget about the diet as you're too tired to make another cup, but the thought of having to wear a swimming costume on your upcoming summer holiday makes you stop. What to do? You'd love to take out a teaspoon of sugar, but you can't. The sugar has been dissolved into the tea.

Do you throw away your tea and go without or is there another way that you could drink this tea knowing that your diet was safe because you've only had one teaspoon of sugar? What about if you only drank half of the cup of tea? You would then be drinking only half of the sugar content, which would be one teaspoon.

The same principle for your cup of tea can be applied to elixirs and ampoules. I have already mentioned that when you give the total volume expressed on the label you will be administering the total weight of the drug specified. Because the weight of the drug has been dissolved in the liquid they have now become intimately linked.

> **? Maths Explained**
>
> In mathematics the weight/volume relationship is referred to as being in proportion to each other. Some of the methods we will be covering using this relationship are known as ratio proportional methods.

This means that whatever you do to the volume, for example take out half or double, the same thing will happen to the drug that is dissolved in it. This is why drinking only half of the volume of tea means that you are having only half of the amount of sugar.

So, for example, using the solution that was 'made' in Figure 8 and shown again in Figure 10: if I were to administer 50ml of this solution, how many grams of the drug would this contain? Remember, that whatever I do to the volume the same thing will happen to the weight: 50ml is half of the volume so this would contain half of the drug weight which in this case is 5 grams. Many drug dosages can be calculated using this method.

Figure 10 A solution containing 10g/100ml

Imagine that I have been told to take 2.5g of the same solution above containing 10g/100ml. How much of the solution should I take? You already know that 50ml would contain 5g so 25ml must contain 2.5g. Therefore I should take 25ml of the solution.

● Halving Method

This method is known as halving (for obvious reasons) and is a useful strategy for calculating weight and volume calculations. The method simply involves halving both the volume and weight until the volume that contains the prescribed dosage is found. As an example let's go back to the question I gave earlier, where your patient needs 5mg of a drug and the stock ampoules contain 20mg/2ml. Using the halving method we can work out the following:

20mg in 2ml   this is the strength of the ampoule
10mg in 1ml   halving dosage and volume
5mg in 0.5ml   halving dosage and volume

Therefore I would administer 0.5ml, which would contain 5mg of the drug.

It is important with weight and volume calculations to always make sure that you understand what it is you are trying to work out and keep this in your mind at all times. For weight and volume calculations, we are trying to work out what volume of the elixir or ampoule contains the prescribed amount.

I know I have mentioned this before, but it is always worth repeating, as it is so important. If at any point during your calculations you are not sure what you are doing, then you need to go back to the question or problem and ensure that you understand what you are trying to do. Without a clear understanding of what you are trying to solve, it is very difficult to make any plans or solve the problem and even more difficult to work out whether your solution is right.

Use the method of halving both the volume and weight to answer the questions in Exercise 9.

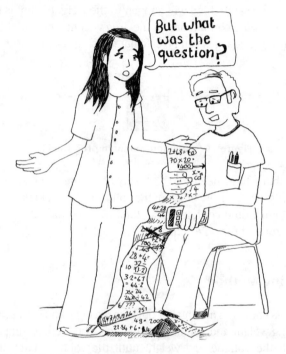

EXERCISE 9

1. Your patient has been prescribed 5mg of a drug. The stock ampoule available contains 10mg in 2ml. How many millilitres do you need to administer?
2. Your patient has been prescribed 75mg of a drug. The stock elixir available contains 150mg in 5ml. How many millilitres do you need to administer?
3. Your patient has been prescribed 125mcg of a drug. The stock ampoules available contain 500mcg in 2ml. How many millilitres do you need to administer?
4. Your patient has been prescribed 50mcg of a drug. The stock syrup available contains 200mcg in 10ml. How many millilitres do you need to administer?
5. Your patient has been prescribed 75mg of a drug. The elixir available contains 50mg in 5ml. How many millilitres do you need to administer?

(Answers: page 220)

The halving method works really well with some dosages of drugs. The dosages that work best with halving are generally those where the amount prescribed is either a half or a quarter of the available dosage on the elixir or ampoule. You can also use halving when the dosage is three-quarters of the available dosage as demonstrated in question five. With three-quarters you can add a half and a quarter together to make three-quarters.

If you are feeling a bit lost here don't worry too much. I have tried to make it even clearer in the maths explained box. I have also given some examples of where you can use the halving method by looking at the dosages you are using in the tips for learning box. However, you can just try this method with each problem and see if you reach the required dosage prescribed when you are repeatedly halving. If you don't reach your prescribed dose then you can know that this method doesn't work for this calculation and try a different method.

? Maths Explained

When you are halving a number you are dividing it by 2. When you halve this number again you can find a quarter of the number, which is effectively dividing the number by 4. For example:

$20 \div 2 = 10 \longrightarrow$ half of $20 = 10 \longrightarrow \frac{1}{2} \times 20 = 10$

$20 \div 4 = 5 \longrightarrow$ quarter of $20 = 5 \longrightarrow \frac{1}{4} \times 20 = 5$

✔ Tips for Learning

Try to become familiar with the common dosages and available dosages in ampoules so you can 'see' immediately what a quarter, three-quarters and a half of these would be:

Dose	Available dose	Fraction	Visualise		
5mg	20mg	Quarter	5mg	15mg	
10mg	20mg	Half	10mg	10mg	
15mg	20mg	Three-quarters	15mg		5mg
25mg	50mg	Half	25mg	25mg	
50mg	100mg	Half	50mg	50mg	
250mg	500mg	Half	250mg	250mg	
500mg	1g or 1000mg	Half	500mg	500mg	

● Doubling

Another method that you can try, using the same principle as before, is known as doubling. No prizes for guessing what this might involve! Earlier, we looked at halving the volume and working out what drug weight this would contain by halving this also. Now we are going to do the same thing but doubling the volume and therefore doubling the drug weight contained as well.

So for example, if you had one ampoule that contained 100mg/1ml, doubling this would give 200mg/2ml. Similarly, if you had an elixir that contains 50mg/2ml, then 4ml would contain double the drug weight, which is 100mg. Hopefully this should seem fairly straightforward. Generally, you will know to try the doubling method when the amount prescribed is greater than the amount in the available ampoule or written on the elixir label.

As you become more experienced you will start to recognise patterns in dosages and will see immediately that a prescribed dose is double or half of the available drug dose. Consider the following example:

Example

A patient who has been prescribed 100mg of a drug and the elixir available contains 50mg/5ml. How many millilitres of the elixir would you administer?

50mg in 5ml   elixir strength available
100mg in 10ml   doubling volume and dosage

You would administer 10ml of the elixir as this will contain 100mg, which is the prescribed dosage.

Now have a go at the following exercise:

EXERCISE 10

1. Your patient requires 500mg of a drug. The elixir available contains 250mg/5ml. How many millilitres of the elixir would you administer?
2. Your patient requires 50mg of a drug. The ampoules available contain 25mg/1ml. How many millilitres would you administer?
3. Your patient requires 20mg of a drug. The suspension available contains 10mg/5ml. How many millilitres would you administer?
4. The available elixir contains 50mg/5ml. You need to administer 200mg. How many millilitres would you administer?
5. You need to administer 20mg to your patient. The suspension available contains 5mg/1ml. How much would you administer?

(Answers: page 220)

To speed up your recognition of number patterns and calculations, it would be useful for you to learn the common numbers and their doubles, halves, quarters. The common numbers found in practice are:

125, 250, 500, 1000

5, 25, 50, 100

20, 40, 60, 80, 100

I have written these so you can begin to see the patterns between these numbers.

So far we have looked at doubling and halving and shown that you can:

- Double and halve the available dosages of ampoules and elixirs until the volume that contains the prescribed dosage we need to administer is found
- Spot patterns in numbers and recognise when a prescribed dosage is a double, half or quarter of the available dose so you know to use doubling or halving methods
- Try doubling and halving without spotting any patterns to see if it helps you to solve the calculation; a trial and error approach
- We have also seen that you can continue doubling or halving the numbers repeatedly until you find the volume containing your prescribed dose

What you can also do with these methods is combine them together. So you may double the volume and also halve it repeatedly and find combinations of volumes and weights, which can help you to solve your calculation. An example is definitely called for here!

Example

Say your patient had been prescribed 125mg of a drug and the elixir contains 50mg/5ml. Now imagine that you haven't recognised any patterns between the dosage prescribed and that available, but you can see that the prescribed dose is greater than that available so you know to start with doubling:

50mg in 5ml   available dose
100mg in 10ml   doubling volume and weight
200mg in 20ml   doubling volume and weight

Quickly you realise that going any further is not going to help you here, but you have found out something useful, and that is that 10ml contains 100mg. If you then go back to your question you want to know how many millilitres would contain 125mg. You now know what volume contains 100mg so you only need to find out what volume contains 25mg and then you can add them together. As 25mg is less than the available dosage of 50mg/5ml I know that I am going to use the halving method now:

50mg in 5ml   available dose
25mg in 2.5ml   halving volume and weight

Now I know that:

125mg = 100mg + 25mg therefore
100mg in 10ml
25mg in 2.5ml
125mg in 10ml + 2.5ml = 12.5ml

You will probably begin to realise that recognising the patterns in the numbers would make calculations like this easier for you, which is why I have suggested that you become familiar with the common numbers used in drug dosages in the tips for learning section. However, you will find that the more you do calculations in practice, the more you will just automatically begin to recognise patterns. For example, with the question above, the expert nurse will look at the 125mg and recognise that this is two and a half times the available dose of 50mg and would immediately know that they need to administer two and a half times 5ml.

EXERCISE 11

1. Your patient requires 600mcg of a drug. The available ampoules contain 400mcg/1ml. How many millilitres would you administer?
2. Your patient has been prescribed 500mg of a drug. The elixir available contains 200mg/2ml. How many millilitres would you administer?
3. Your patient has been prescribed 50mg of a drug. The elixir available contains 20mg/1ml. How many millilitres would you administer?
4. The available ampoules contain 40mg/1ml. You need to administer 60mg to your patient. How many millilitres would you administer?
5. You need to administer 150mcg of a drug to your patient. The available ampoules contain 60mcg/1ml. How many millilitres would you administer?

(Answers: page 220)

For some dosages, however, the halving and doubling methods don't work. This is generally where the dose prescribed is not a half or a quarter of the available dose and so doubling and halving is not useful. For example, if a patient was prescribed 3mg of a drug and the available dosage for this drug was 10mg/2ml and you tried the halving method:

10mg in 2ml
5mg in 1ml
2.5mg in 0.5ml

This information is not helpful. This is when you need to use a different method.

✔ Tips for Learning

The halving method can be useful to estimate what volume you would expect to administer. For instance, using the example above you have found out that 5mg is contained in 1ml and 2.5mg is contained in 0.5ml. As 3mg is between 5mg and 2.5mg, you can expect the volume you need to administer to be between 0.5ml and 1ml, but closer to 0.5ml as 2.5mg is closer to 3mg than 5mg.

● Reducing Down to a Single Unit

Another method that you could try is based on the same principle as before that the volume and weight are proportional, but instead of doubling and halving, this time you work out what volume contains a single unit of drug weight.

So you may try to work out what volume contains 10mg or 1mg because you can then use this information to calculate most other dosages. For example, if I know what volume contains 1mg of the drug then I can work out 6mg by multiplying the volume by six, or if 3mg, by multiplying this volume by three.

Similarly, if your prescribed dosage is a multiple of 10, such as 20mg or 30mg, then you can work out what volume contains 10mg and multiply this volume by either two or three to find out what volume contains your prescribed dose.

To reduce the weight of the drug down to single units you usually need to divide the volume and weight by 10 or 100.

Using the example from before, you need to give 3mg of a drug and the ampoule contains 10mg/2ml. Using the reducing down to single units method, we would divide the volume and the weight by 10:

10mg in 2ml   available dose
1mg in 0.2ml   dividing volume and weight by 10

Now we know that 0.2ml contains 1mg. We need three lots of 1mg to give the prescribed dose of 3mg, so we need three lots of the 0.2ml volume:

3mg in 0.6ml   multiplying by 3

Therefore the prescribed dose of 3mg is contained in 0.6ml.

Example

Imagine that your patient has been prescribed 20mcg and the elixir contains 100mcg/5ml. Using the reducing down to single units method, you would be aiming to work out what volume contains 10mcg and then multiply this by 2 to give the volume that contains 20mcg:

100mcg in 5ml   available dose
10mcg in 0.5ml   dividing volume and weight by 10
20mcg in 1ml   multiplying volume and weight by 2

So 1ml of this elixir would contain 20mcg.

EXERCISE 12

1.   Your patient has been prescribed 6mg of a drug. The ampoules available contain 10mg/1ml. How many millilitres would you administer?

2. Your patient has been prescribed 40mcg of a drug. The elixir available contains 100mcg/5ml. How many millilitres would you administer?
3. Your patient has been prescribed 30mg of a drug. The ampoules available contain 100mg/2ml. How many millilitres would you administer?
4. The available elixir contains 100mg/2ml. You need to administer 60mg to your patient. How many millilitres would you administer?
5. You need to administer 2mg of drug to a patient. Using the available elixir of 10mg/10ml, work out how many millilitres you should administer.

(Answers: page 220)

Now you have learnt three methods for solving weight and volume calculations:

- Halving
- Doubling
- Reducing down to a single unit

What you can now do is use a combination of all three of these methods to solve calculations that are not as straightforward as the questions I have given you so far. For example, if the available dose is not already in tens or hundreds then you can use the doubling and halving method to work out a weight that is either a ten or a hundred and then reduce down to the single unit. For example, if a patient was prescribed 20mg and the available dose was 50mg/2ml:

50mg in 2ml	available dose
100mg in 4ml	doubling
10mg in 0.4ml	reduce to single unit
20mg in 0.8ml	multiplying by 2

With these three methods it is mostly trial and error to start with, playing around with the numbers until the required dosage is worked out. As you become more practised and experienced at these calculations, though, you will be able to recognise the relationship between the prescribed dose and available dose and select the best method to use.

✔ Tips for Learning

If prescribed dose is less than available dose:
- Start with halving method
- If halving method unsuccessful, make a note of estimate for answer
- Try reducing down to single units

- Double or halve dosages to give ten or hundred as a weight before reducing to single unit if necessary

If prescribed dose is more than available dose:
- Start with doubling method
- If doubling unsuccessful, take away what volume and dosage is known from the prescribed dose to find out what you still need to work out. For example, if prescribed 125mg and elixir available is 100mg/5ml, take away 100mg from 125mg to leave 25mg which you still need to work out the volume for
- Use halving method
- If unsuccessful, use reducing down to single units as above

Relationships

The methods we have been using so far rely on manipulation of the volume and weight until the volume that contains the desired dosage is found. I have already indicated that recognition of the relationship between the dosage prescribed and the available dose can help you to plan what method would work best.

For example, if the dosage prescribed was 25mg and the available dose was 100mg/2ml, then knowing that 25mg is a quarter of 100mg will help you to choose halving as an appropriate method to use. Similarly, if you recognise that a prescribed dose of 250mg is double the available 125mg/5ml elixir, then you can chose the doubling method immediately as an appropriate method.

Once you become more adept at recognising the relationships between the numbers in prescribed dosages and those in available dosages, then you can use this knowledge to work out the volume to administer without manipulating the numbers.

Recognition of the relationship between numbers still relies on the same principle that the weight and volume in elixirs and ampoules are proportionate, but uses the relationship between the prescribed dose and available dose to work out what *part* of the available dose to administer.

? Maths Explained

The part of the available dose that we wish to administer, out of the total dose available, is really asking 'what part of the whole dose do I need to administer?' This is the same as asking 'what fraction of this total dose do I need to administer?' We are actually dealing with fractions here.

Once you know what part of the weight you need to administer, then you know that you need to administer the same part of the volume because whatever you do to the weight, you also do to the volume.

Let me give you an example that has been mentioned already. Imagine your patient has been prescribed 5mg and the available ampoule contains 20mg/2ml. Before, we halved the available dose until we were able to see that 5mg/0.5ml.

But equally I could look at the prescribed dose of 5mg and know that this is one quarter of 20mg so I need to administer one quarter of 2ml, which would be 0.5ml. I have tried to represent this relationship in the diagram in Box 11.

Box 11	**Visual representation of relationship between prescribed dose and available dose**

Prescribed dose is 5mg

5mg	5mg
5mg	5mg

0.5ml	0.5ml
0.5ml	0.5ml

20mg   in   2ml

✔ Tips for Learning

It would be useful to be able to recognise the common relationships between the prescribed doses and the available dose of the medicine. I have summarised the most useful relationships here.

Prescribed dose	Available dose	Relationship
5mg	10mg	half
10mg	20mg	half
50mg	100mg	half
5mg	20mg	quarter
25mg	100mg	quarter
15mg	20mg	three-quarters
20mg	50mg	two-fifths
2mg	10mg	fifth
2mg	5mg	two-fifths

Prescribed dose	Available dose	Relationship
8mg	10mg	four-fifths
1mg	10mg	tenth
0.1mg	1mg	tenth

Sometimes it is easier to visualise these relationships by looking at a syringe:

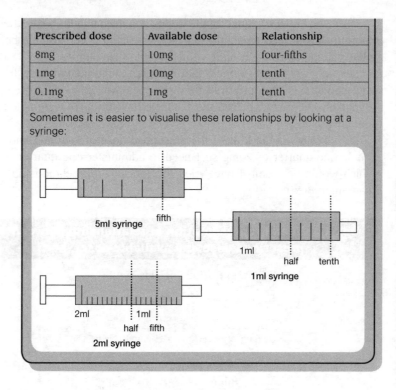

Let's look at another example where the relationship between the prescribed dose and available dose is examined first. Say your patient has been prescribed 10mg and the available dose is 20mg/1ml. Using the relationship method, you would see that 10mg is one half of 20mg so you need to administer half of the volume, which would be 0.5ml (see Figure 11).

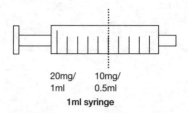

Figure 11 A visual representation of 10mg/0.5ml

This isn't really much different from the halving method except that you are thinking in a slightly different way and using the dosage you require, that is, 10mg as your starting point rather than an ending point! In other words, you are thinking 'what do I need to do to 10mg in order to get 20mg?'

Now for a slightly more difficult example, imagine that your patient has been prescribed 20mg and the available suspension is 50mg/2ml.

So starting with the 20mg what relationship is this to the 50mg? This is obviously where your clinical experience and knowledge of numbers come in handy. Ten would be one-fifth of 50mg so 20mg is two-fifths of 50mg.

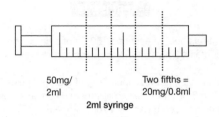

50mg/
2ml

Two fifths =
20mg/0.8ml

2ml syringe

Figure 12 Visual representation of 50mg in 2ml

You now know that you need to administer two-fifths of the available weight so this is the same as two-fifths of the volume, which is 0.8ml (use Figure 12 to help visualise this). Use Exercise 13 to practise this method.

✔ Tips for Learning

When you have a dosage that is in 2ml of volume, it is sometimes easier to either visualise a 2ml syringe to calculate the dosage or work out the dosage as if it is 1ml and then double this. For example, if you have worked out that you need to administer two-fifths of the 2ml ampoule you can visualise this as two lots of 1ml, so one-fifth would be 0.2ml. You can visualise this by looking at the syringes illustrated below. If one-fifth is 0.2ml, then two-fifths will be double this and be 0.4ml. Remember that this is for 1ml and you want two-fifths of 2ml so you need 0.4ml again to make 0.8ml.

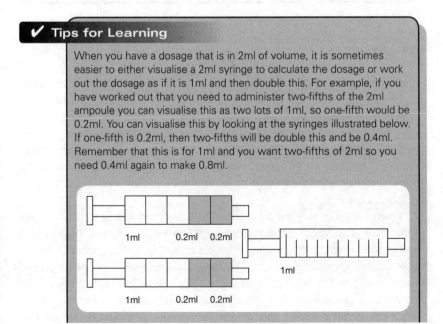

1ml   0.2ml   0.2ml

1ml

1ml   0.2ml   0.2ml

Each measurement of a 1ml syringe will be 0.1ml (1ml divided into 10 parts will be 0.1ml), so two measurements would be 0.2ml. If you count up every two measurements, you will see that there are five lots of 0.2, so 0.2ml is one-fifth of 1ml. Two-fifths of 1ml will therefore be 0.4ml and two-fifths of 2ml will be two-fifths of 1ml twice to give 0.8ml.

EXERCISE 13

1. Your patient has been prescribed 150mg of a drug. The suspension available contains 200mg/10ml. How many millilitres would you administer?
2. Your patient has been prescribed 2mg of a drug. The ampoule available contains 6mg/3ml. How many millilitres would you administer?
3. Your patient has been prescribed 20mcg of a drug. The elixir available contains 100mcg/5ml. How many millilitres would you administer?
4. The available ampoule contains 5mg/2ml. You need to administer 3mg. How many millilitres would you administer?
5. You need to administer 80mg of a drug. The available ampoule contains 100mg/2ml. How many millilitres would you administer?

(Answers: page 220)

● **Syringes**

I have already mentioned how you can use syringes to help you with calculations in one of the tips for learning, but it is worth spending some more time on this, since syringes are such a useful tool. When you are measuring elixirs and drawing up volumes to administer as injections, syringes are the most frequent and accurate tools that we tend to use to measure the volume required. Because of this many nurses use syringes not only to measure, but to also calculate the volume to be administered and as a check that this volume is correct.

I have only become aware recently of how important a tool this is for some nurses and how difficult solving calculations are if this tool is taken away from them, for example in a classroom setting. I once asked a colleague to undertake a written calculation assessment for me as part of some research I was undertaking on calculations before I realised the importance of syringes. My colleague relied on syringes as her method to solve calculations and so laboriously drew syringes for each question so she could work out the solution! Since then I always make sure that I have syringes available when I am teaching or assessing!

Not all syringes have the numerical label for each measurement on the side. For example, the 2ml syringe will only have the labels for 1ml and 2ml written next to the measurements. This means that as nurses we need to know and be able to work out what measurement each mark on the syringe refers to. To do this you need to count the number of measurements and divide the syringe volume by this number. The answer will tell you what volume each measurement refers to. For example, using the 2ml syringe there are 20 measurements marked on the syringe (up to the 2ml measurement; 2ml syringes do have measurements up to 2.5ml). Dividing 2ml by 20 gives 0.1, so each mark refers to 0.1ml. It is useful to become familiar and learn what the different volume measurements refer to on each syringe (see Figure 13).

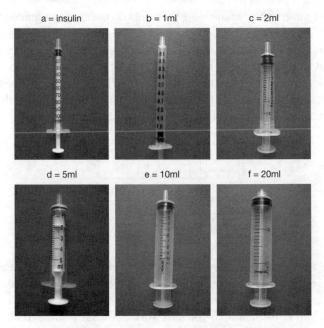

Figure 13 Common syringes used in healthcare

✔ **Tips for Learning**

When drawing up liquid in a syringe, it is important that you are aware of how to ensure the correct volume is measured. Some syringes have a rubber component that helps to draw up the liquid, which can make measuring tricky. You need to remember that you are ensuring that the liquid in your syringe contains the exact volume required. Air bubbles or the wrong part of the syringe plunger used as the measurement can result in the patient receiving a smaller dose than prescribed. The syringe in this diagram shows where measurements need to be taken from:

1ml

1ml syringe

Bottom of syringe plunger
ensures that there is 0.5ml of
volume measured

With syringes you use the measurements on the side as a guide to calculate the drug dosage. So for example, if you had an available dose of 10mg/1ml you would use a 2ml syringe and use the measurements to work out what weight of the drug each measurement would be. If you look at the 1ml syringe in Figure 14 you can see that the 1ml is divided into ten measurements. You can use this to divide the dose by 10 to work out that each measurement on the syringe contains 1mg of the drug.

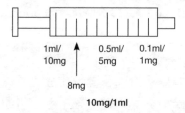

1ml/   0.5ml/   0.1ml/
10mg   5mg   1mg

8mg

10mg/1ml

Figure 14 A 1ml syringe showing the measurements and dosage of a 10mg/ml strength solution and indicating the volume containing an 8mg dose

Once you know this then you can work out what volume to administer of any dosage that is prescribed. For example, 2mg would be two measurements of the syringe and 8mg would be eight measurements. This is why some nurses find it difficult to state the *number* of millilitres to administer, because they have used the syringe and don't necessarily need to state what the volume is. If you prefer to be able to state exactly what volume you are administering (and ideally you should be able to do this), then you need to divide the volume by the number of measurements. For a 1ml syringe each measurement represents 0.1ml.

Use the syringe in Figure 14 to work out the answers to the questions in Exercise 14:

EXERCISE 14

1. Your patient has been prescribed 6mg of a drug. The ampoules available contain 10mg/1ml. How many millilitres would you administer?
2. Your patient has been prescribed 20mg of a drug. The ampoules available contain 50mg in 1ml. How many millilitres would you administer?
3. Your patient has been prescribed 20mcg of a drug. The ampoules available contain 50mcg/2ml. How many millilitres would you administer?
4. The ampoules available contain 50mg/2ml. You need to administer 30mg, how many millilitres would you administer?
5. You need to administer 15mg of a drug. The ampoules available contain 25mg/2ml. How much would you administer?

(Answers: page 221)

● **Prefilled Syringes**

Some drugs are manufactured in syringes which have been prefilled with a set dosage of the drug. The needle on the syringe has been designed so that it can be given at 90 degrees subcutaneously. The manufacturers of prefilled syringes advise that air bubbles are not dispelled before administering to avoid loss of the drug. A common example of prefilled syringes is the low molecular weight heparins such as Clexane.

Warning!
Calculations may still be required with prefilled syringes, however, and it may be that only a part of the prefilled syringe needs to be administered. For example, some dosages of heparins are prescribed according to the person's body weight, so the patient may need a specific amount from a

syringe, such as requiring 9000IU from a prefilled syringe containing 10 000IU/ml. In this example you need to work out how much of the volume in the syringe would contain 9000IU. This is a weight volume calculation, which we have just covered. In this case you would administer 0.9ml from the syringe.

The Nursing Formula

You may have been wondering when I was going to mention the 'nursing formula' and whether I had forgotten to include it. I haven't forgotten the formula method, but have deliberately placed it last in the list of potential methods.

The most important part of solving a drug calculation is understanding what the calculation or problem is asking you to do. Until you are clear about this, you cannot start planning or solving the calculation and cannot examine your solution to decide whether it is a realistic and appropriate solution to the problem presented.

The formula method does not encourage understanding. So before you start using this method, I wanted to get you thinking logically about what calculation questions are asking you and using some of the methods that allow you to 'see' clearly the steps you are taking to solve the problem.

There are many problems with the formula method (Wright, 2008):

- You can use it without clearly understanding what it is you are doing. This also means that you can obtain solutions that you don't fully understand
- Nurses seem to switch off their logical brain when they are using the formula method. I have observed experienced nurses in a classroom using the formula to work out how much to administer if the patient needed 10mg and the ampoules contain 20mg/2ml
- You can 'learn' how to solve written drug calculations using the formula and produce answers without understanding what you are doing. This understanding is vital so you can be sure your answer is right and pick up errors
- The formula can be used incorrectly, giving the wrong solution. The unclear understanding of the drug calculation means that these errors can be missed

The formula method does, however, have a place in drug calculations:

- When the dosages that you are working with do not have nice straightforward relationships like doubles or halves or when doubling, halving or reducing down to single units can be more complicated and time consuming. This is particularly the case in clinical areas where you are using the weights of the patients to calculate initial dosages so you don't have nice easy numbers to deal with
- When you are tired or are pressured and you need to work out the dosage really quickly
- As another useful method for checking calculations. Some nurses prefer to use the formula method and then use other methods such as doubling and halving to check that the answer is correct

---

Warning!
As long as you understand what it is you are doing and think logically about your solution using this understanding, then the formula is a useful method. Without this understanding, the formula method can do more harm than good.

Having gone on at length, giving tales of doom and gloom about the formula method, it probably would be a good idea to tell you what it is for those that don't know.

The formula method is basically using a mathematical formula that takes you through the calculation without your having to think about what you are doing. With the formula, you place the numbers of the dosages and volume involved in the problem you are trying to solve into the formula, to set up your calculation.

Once you have your calculation set up, you can then solve this to arrive at your answer. You then need to translate your answer back to the original question so you know what this 'number' you have arrived at actually means. Your numerical answer is the volume that you need to administer of the ampoule or suspension that you are dealing with.

Nursing Formula is:

$$\frac{\textbf{what you want}}{\textbf{what you have available}} \times \text{volume it's in} = \text{volume to administer}$$

? Maths Explained

The formula is actually the same method as the relationship method above, but formalised so that you can use it with numbers where you can't see a relationship easily. The formula is asking the same question though – what relationship is the dosage I need to give to the dosage available? – that is, what part it is of the whole. Once I know that, I just do the same to the volume and take the same part of that volume.

For example, if I needed to administer 8mg from a 20mg/2ml ampoule, I am actually trying to find out what fraction 8mg is of 20mg so that I can draw up the same fraction of volume. This is the same as saying 8mg out of a possible 20mg, which is $8/20$. I therefore need eight-twentieths of the 2ml volume:

$8/20 \times 2 = 2/5 \times 2 = 0.4$ml

Can you see that this is the same as the formula?

✔ Tips for Learning

If you were using a calculator and the formula method for the example in maths explained above, you would key in:

$\boxed{8}\boxed{\div}\boxed{2}\boxed{0}\boxed{\times}\boxed{2}\boxed{=}$

The first step then if you are going to use the formula method is having some way of remembering this formula. You will hear nurses chanting 'what I want, over what I have multiplied by what it's in' as a way of remembering the formula. Other people find this difficult to remember and need to actually write down the formula, which they keep with them at all times when in clinical practice.

You need to find a reliable way of ensuring you remember the formula for yourself if this is a method that you want to use. It is very common for nurses to remember the formula incorrectly and think that it is what you have available over what you want. This obviously gives a very different answer! So finding time to work out a way of always remembering this formula is not time wasted!

✔ Tips for Learning

To help you remember the order of the formula you can shorten it to WHI (pronounced 'wee') which stands for Want, Have, In and could help you to remember that it is:

W/H × I

Alternatively, the formula actually follows the order that you would
follow in clinical practice, that is, you would look at the patient's
medicine chart to find out what is 'wanted', then you would go to the
patient's locker or stock cupboard to find the elixir/ampoule and find out
'what you have' and 'what it's in'. If you are doing calculations in a
classroom setting and can't remember the formula, it may be useful for
you to visualise what you would do in clinical practice to help
remember the formula order.

With the formula method, you need to develop the skills of selecting the
information that the formula is asking for, either from clinical practice, that
is, a medicine chart and solution, or, if a written question, from carefully
reading the question. So you need to know:

- What dosage the patient has been prescribed
- The dosage of the available solution
- The volume of the ampoule

These pieces of information are then placed into the formula as directed
to set up the calculation. Let me give an example to make this clearer. You
need to give 124mg of gentamicin. The ampoules available are 40mg/ml.
How many millilitres would you administer? I will work through this question below:

$$\frac{\text{what you want}}{\text{what you have available}} \times \text{what it's in} = \text{volume to administer}$$

what you want = 124mg
what you have available is 40mg
what it's in = 1ml

So my calculation will be:

$$\frac{124\text{mg}}{40\text{mg}} \times 1\text{ml} = \text{volume to administer}$$

Now you have this calculation set up, the tricky bit and the bit that
causes lots of difficulties is the solving of it. If you are using a calculator,
then it is fairly straightforward because you just have to put the numbers
into the calculator and it will give you the numerical answer. (See maths
explained if unsure how to put this formula into a calculator.)

If you are not using a calculator, then you will need to use some of your arithmetic skills in order to solve it. To make this calculation easier, you will need to be able to reduce the fraction to its lowest value and/or then do long division.

> **? Maths Explained**
>
> If you are unsure about how to do this or why we should even do this, then please refer to the section that explains this in Chapter 4.

With this example, you can see from the working out below that I have reduced the fraction $^{124}\!/_{40}$ to smaller numbers by dividing the top and bottom number by 2 (often termed as 'cancelling down'). This gave $^{62}\!/_{20}$. I did the same thing again as both numbers are still even so I know that they are divisible by 2 to get $^{31}\!/_{10}$.

At this point I can do two things:

1. I can either go into long division to work out what 31 is divided by 10. (The working out for long division is shown in Box 12.)
2. Or I can use my knowledge of multiplying and dividing by 10 which we did in Chapter 1 when we covered converting between units of measurement to work out that $31 \div 10$ is 3.1 by moving the decimal place one place (or moving the number down the number line).

Box 12   Long division procedure for the sum 31 divided by 10

$$\begin{array}{r} 0\,3.\,1 \\ 10\,\overline{)3\,1._10\,0} \end{array}$$

The procedure and thought process is:

(a)   10 into 3 can't go, so carry the 3 to make 31
(b)   10 into 31 goes 3, remainder 1. Put the answer 3 above and carry the 1 to make 10
(c)   10 into 10 goes 1. Put the answer 1 above
(d)   The answer to 31 divided by 10 is 3.1 (this is explained in more detail in Chapter 4 so don't worry too much if you have not followed this long division procedure)

Because the formula has so many little operations to it, when you don't use a calculator the potential for error increases also. This means that you need to be especially vigilant when checking your processes. Ideally you should check each part of your calculation before you move on to the next part. For example, check that you've reduced your fraction down correctly before you move on to long division. I have given three more worked examples below to help you to become familiar with this method.

Examples

1. Your patient has been prescribed 2mg of a drug. The ampoules available contain 6mg/3ml. How many millilitres would you administer?

$$\frac{\text{what you want}}{\text{what you have available}} \times \text{what it's in}$$

$$\frac{2}{6} \times 3 = \text{volume to administer}$$

Reduce fractions down either by dividing 6 and 3 by 3 (option 1 below) or by dividing 2 and 6 by 2 (option 2 below).

Option 1

$$\frac{2}{2} \times 1 = 1$$

Option 2

$$\frac{1}{3} \times 3 = 3 = 1$$

2. Your patient requires 170mcg of a drug. The suspension contains 200mcg/5ml. How many millilitres would you administer?

$$\frac{\text{what you want}}{\text{what you have available}} = \text{volume to administer}$$

$$\frac{170}{200} \times 5 = \text{volume to administer}$$

Reduce fractions down by either dividing 170mg and 200mcg by 10 to get 17mg over 20mcg and then dividing the 20mcg and 5ml by 5 (option 1 below) or by dividing 5ml and 200ml by 5 to get 40mg and 1ml and then dividing 170mg and 40mg by 10 (option 2 below).

Option 1

$$\frac{17}{20} \times 5 = \frac{17}{4} \times 1$$

Option 2

$$\frac{170}{40} \times 1 = \frac{17}{4}$$

With both options you have reduced your calculation to easier numbers and now need to use long division to divide 17 by 4:

$$
\begin{array}{r}
0\,4.\,2\;5 \\
4\,\overline{\big|\,1\;7.{}_{1}0\;{}_{2}0\;0\;0}
\end{array}
$$

= 4.25ml to administer

3.   Your patient has been prescribed 45mg of a drug. The ampoules available contain 100mg/2ml. How many millilitres would you administer?

$$\frac{\text{what you want}}{\text{what you have available}} \times \text{what it's in} = \text{volume to administer}$$

$$\frac{45}{100} \times 2$$

Reduce fractions down either by dividing 45 and 100 by 5 to get 9 over 20 and then divide 2 and the 20 by 2 (option 1) or divide 100 and 2 by 2 to get 50 and 1 and then divide the 45 and 50 by 5 to get 9 over 20 (option 2).

Option 1

$$\frac{9}{20} \times 2 = \frac{18}{20} = \frac{9}{10} = 0.9\text{ml}$$

Option 2

$$\frac{45}{50} \times 1 = \frac{45}{50} = \frac{9}{10} = 0.9\text{ml}$$

Hopefully you have followed all these examples okay and they make sense to you. The main thing with formula calculations when you are not using a calculator is to keep practising them so that you become more confident at reducing down fractions, multiplying fractions and long division. The more you practise the easier it will become, honest!

This is a good time to remind you again about checking your answer, especially important if you are using the formula method, to be absolutely certain that you have arrived at the correct answer. In Box 5 (see Chapter 1), I went through the different methods you could use to check your solutions. If you can't remember these, please take some time to revise them and ensure you get into the habit of using some of these methods.

Using some of these checking methods, have a look at the questions and solutions in Exercise 15 and identify whether the solutions are correct. Try to complete this without actually doing the calculations yourself. For each question, try to give a clear rationale as to why this solution is right or wrong. Imagine you are double-checking a drug calculation and the nurse you are checking with is adamant that their solution is correct.

EXERCISE 15

1. Your patient has been prescribed 250mg of amoxicillin. The suspension available contains 125mg/5ml.
   Solution – administer 2.5ml
2. Your patient requires 6mg hyoscine. The ampoules available contain 400mcg/ml.
   Solution – administer 15ml
3. You need to administer 5mg morphine. The ampoules available contain 20mg/ml.
   Solution – administer 0.25ml
4. You need to administer 15 000 units of a heparin. The ampoules available contain 25 000 units/ml
   Solution – administer 0.8ml
5. You need to administer 150mg of phenytoin. The suspension available contains 30mg/5ml.
   Solution – 25ml

(Answers: page 221)

Warning!
It is really important if you are using the formula and not using a calculator that you always keep in your mind what it is that you are trying to work out. When you have to do so many different arithmetic operations such as reducing fractions, multiplying fractions, long division and so on, you can easily lose the plot and what it is you are actually trying to do. If you ever feel like you've forgotten what you are trying to do, then just stop and go back to the question you are trying to solve and ensure you understand it again.

I have added some practice questions for you here to help you to become familiar with the calculation skills required, or with using the formula. I have separated each skill out so that you can practise each in turn and ensure you are happy with these before moving on or can practise only the skill that you feel less confident on.

If you find these questions too difficult or are not sure you understand what you are doing, then you may wish to go to the section on fractions and long division in Chapter 4. For those of you who feel confident with multiplication of fractions, reducing down and long division, then you can skip right past this section!

EXERCISE 16

Calculate the following:
1. $100/20 \times 1$
2. $50/5 \times 2$
3. $100/50 \times 5$
4. $5/20 \times 2$
5. $500/250 \times 2$

Reduce the following fractions to the lowest numbers:
1. $125/100$
2. $12/48$
3. $75/125$
4. $30/150$
5. $45/10$

Express the following fractions as decimals (long division):
1. $15/2$
2. $3/5$
3. $7/35$
4. $45/4$
5. $172/8$

(Answers: page 221)

You should now be feeling fairly confident with using the formula and completing the calculation you set up with this method without a calculator. For the exercise below, you can choose whether you do these calculations with a calculator or using your arithmetic skills or do some of each.

Warning!
In practice, it is common for nurses to use a calculator to solve drug calculations and this is fine provided that you always have a calculator with you. The difficulty occurs when you have to solve a calculation and do not have a calculator available or you have to complete a drug calculation test without using a calculator.

Some nurse educators and regulatory bodies such as the NMC (Nursing and Midwifery Council) in the UK recommend that calculators should not be a substitute for arithmetic skills such as the long division, multiplication and fractions you have been practising, so it is worth ensuring that you are confident at these skills if you are going to use the formula method.

Like all skills, if you don't use them you will lose them! So, even if you prefer using a calculator, you need to keep your arithmetic skills alive by regularly solving the calculation without a calculator.

Do this regularly and you'll keep these arithmetic skills finely tuned and you never know, you may even start to enjoy them!

? Maths Explained

Useful sections that could help you with these calculations are multiplying and dividing by multiples of 10 and multiplying fractions. These are explained in Chapter 4 and I would recommend if you are a little unsure that you take some time out to look at these areas to ensure you are confident.

✔ Tips for Learning

You can recognise what numbers are divisible by other numbers by using some rules. These are:
- Numbers divisible by 2 are always even
- Numbers divisible by 10 always end in a zero
- Numbers divisible by 5 always end in a 5 or a zero

EXERCISE 17

1. Your patient requires 35mg of a drug. The ampoules available are 50mg/2ml. How many millilitres would you administer?

2.   Your patient has been prescribed 150 units of a drug. The ampoules contain 1000 units/1ml. How many millilitres would you administer?

3.   Your patient has been prescribed 60mg of a drug. The suspension available is 150mg/5ml. How many millilitres would you administer?

4.   You need to give you patient 120mcg of a drug. The suspension available contains 500mcg/5ml. How many millilitres would you administer?

5.   The suspension available is 250mg/5ml. You need to give 600mg. How many millilitres would you administer?

(Answers: page 222)

Warning!
The method that you choose to solve drug calculations doesn't really matter as long as you understand what you are doing and can explain how you reached this answer to someone else. This is especially important if you work in clinical areas that have a policy which involves two nurses checking drug calculations with both needing to sign to say that the calculation and drug dosage to be administered is correct. In these situations you both need to be completely sure that your answer is correct. You should never agree with another nurse's calculation if you don't understand or are not sure that their calculation is correct. Remember that you are both equally responsible and accountable for the drug administration.

I have covered quite a few different methods for solving weight and volume calculations and have given you exercises for each method where you could practise trying them out. I have also mentioned that it doesn't really matter which method you use as long as you feel comfortable and confident with this method. From my observation of nurses solving calculations, though, I have become aware that nurses will often chose a method which best suits the question being asked rather than stick to one method for all questions.

Obviously the knowledge of which method to use will be developed with experience and for now it is fine for you to have only two methods that you prefer to use. It is worth keeping an open mind, though, and considering using a range of methods as your confidence and clinical experience develop so you have the possibility of adapting your calculation methods to suit the calculation and the situation.

So far I have separated the different methods for solving weight/volume calculations and given exercises to solve using only the method we were discussing. To help you begin to develop the skills of matching the calculation method with particular calculations, I have given you an exercise here.

If you are still feeling a little overwhelmed and feel safer sticking to one method you prefer, then please by all means stick to that method to solve these. For others who are feeling more confident and daring, look at the numbers involved in the calculation and use these as a guide for deciding on the calculation method.

EXERCISE 18

1. Your patient has been prescribed 42mg. The elixir available is 50mg/5ml. What volume of the elixir would you administer?
2. You need to give 50mg of a drug. The drug ampoule strength is 200mg/2ml. What volume of the ampoule do you need to draw up?
3. Your patient has been prescribed 30mg of a drug. The drug elixir strength is 20mg/2ml. How much of the elixir would you administer to the patient?
4. Your patient requires 250mg of a drug. The elixir contains 100mg/5ml. What volume would you administer?
5. You need to administer 80mg of a drug to a patient. The ampoules available are 100mg/5ml. How many millilitres (ml) would you administer from this ampoule?

(Answers: page 222)

● **Complex Questions using Weight and Volume**

So far we have concentrated on the different methods you can use to solve weight and volume calculations and given lots of exercises to help you become familiar and confident with these different methods. The next step is to combine some of the other methods that you learnt and practised in Chapter 1 with these weight and volume calculations.

Calculations involving weight and volume may also require you to calculate the dosage required for the individual patient first and also convert the units of measurements involved so that both the prescribed and available dosages are expressed in the same units of measurements. For example, your patient may have been prescribed 200mcg/kg and the available ampoules may be available as 1mg/2ml. Here you will have to carry out several steps in order to solve the calculation.

As I mentioned in Chapter 1, it is really important that initially you carry out each step of the calculation until you become more familiar and confident with these calculations (see Box 13).

Box 13   Step by step guide to solving weight volume calculations

1. Make sure you understand the question and what exactly you are trying to work out: for example dosage for the individual patient and then how much of the available drug to give in order to administer this dosage.

2. Calculate the individual dose for the patient by multiplying their weight in kilograms by the dosage per kilogram.

3. Go back to the question and check that you are still clear about your understanding. For example: I know the actual dosage, I now need to calculate how much of the available drug to administer.

4. Check that the prescribed dosage has the same unit of measurements as the available drug dosage.

5. If the units of measurement are different, then convert the prescribed dosage so it is expressed in the same unit of measurement as the available drug.

6. Go back to the question and check that you are still clear about your understanding. For example: I need to administer this dosage, I have this dosage available and they are both now in the same unit of measurement. I now need to work out what volume of this suspension, elixir or ampoule would give the prescribed dosage.

7. Examine the dosages in the question and decide which method would be best to solve the calculation. If you are unsure, start with doubling and halving or use the formula method.

8. Work out how much of the available drug to administer by using your chosen methods.

9. Check your answer makes sense in relation to the questions and the dosages being prescribed and available, and your knowledge of clinical practice. For example, does it seem reasonable to administer this amount of a drug? Have I ever administered this amount before? Is this the usual volume that I administer for this particular drug?

10. If you are unsure, check through your work or use a different method. If you are still unsure, you need to ask for help.

EXERCISE 19

1. Your patient has been prescribed 2mg/kg gentamicin as an IM injection. Your patient weighs 72kg and the ampoules available are 40mg/ml. How many millilitres of this ampoule strength would you need to administer?

2. You need to administer 5mg/kg phenytoin to your patient in two divided doses orally. The suspension available is 30mg/5ml. Your patient's weight is 16.8kg. How many millilitres would you administer for each dose?

3. The prescription for your patient is for 3g amoxicillin every 12 hours orally. You need to give the first dose of this drug to your patient. The suspension available is 250mg/5ml. How many millilitres do you need to administer?

4. Your patient has been prescribed 1.5mg/kg frusemide orally. The paediatric liquid available is 1mg/1ml. How many millilitres would you need to administer to your patient, who weighs 4kg?

5. You need to administer 0.25mg digoxin to your patient. The elixir available contains 50mcg/ml. How many millilitres do you need to administer?

(Answers: page 222)

Millimoles

Some drug strengths are expressed as the number of moles or millimoles that are contained in a set volume of liquid (see Box 2, in Chapter 1). Calculations involving millimoles or moles are solved in the same way as weight/volume calculations. For example, a baby is prescribed 4mmols of potassium to be added to an infusion and the potassium ampoules available contain 20mmol/10ml. In this example you need to calculate how many millilitres of the potassium ampoule contain 4mmols. Can you see that this is no different from the calculations we have been doing using weight/volume and would be calculated in the same way:

Doubling/halving and single units

20mmol	10ml
10mmol	5ml
2mmol	1ml
4mmol	2ml

Relationship – recognising that 4mmol is a fifth of 20mmol ($4 \times 5 = 20$mmol) so you need one-fifth of 10ml, which is 2ml.

Formula

$$\frac{4\text{mmol}}{20\text{mmol}} \times 10\text{ml} = 2\text{ml}$$

Reconstituting

Sometimes drugs are manufactured in an ampoule in a powder form. These drugs are unstable in a liquid form, which means their properties may change and so they have to be 'made' into a liquid before they can be administered. Due to the unstable nature of these drugs, they must be used soon after they are placed into a liquid.

Generally, drugs that are manufactured in a powder form need 'reconstituting' with water or sodium chloride before they can be administered. The type of liquid recommended for reconstituting drugs is written on the information accompanying the drug and should be checked before the drug is reconstituted. The most common drugs that are manufactured in a powder form and require reconstituting are intravenous drugs such as antibiotics.

Warning!

When reconstituting drugs, the volume added to the ampoule increases as the drug 'displaces' some of the volume. (You can see this effect when you get into a bath; your body 'displaces' some of the water and the volume of the bath appears more.) As a result, the volume that you add becomes slightly more once the drug has been reconstituted. This is such a small disparity that it usually makes little difference to the overall calculation. However, when dealing with very small dosages, such as in caring for neonates, this displacement volume can make a difference and therefore needs to be accounted for. Each specific drug has a displacement volume calculated – that is, the amount of volume that is 'displaced' through the reconstituting of a set amount of the drug. This displacement volume needs to be subtracted from the volume you are going to add to the ampoule.

For example, a 250mg amoxicillin vial has a displacement volume of 0.2ml. To make up a solution of 250mg/5ml, I would need to reconstitute with 5ml minus the displacement volume of 0.2ml. This would be 4.8ml. Once reconstituted, the volume will be 250mg/5ml as the drug has displaced the volume in the same way that your body does in the bath. Information about specific displacement values for each drug can be found in clinical areas where displacement needs to be accounted for.

In the powder form the drug dosage is expressed in weight only, so there may be an ampoule of benzylpenicillin which has the dosage of 600mg. However, once you have reconstituted the drug with a liquid, it then has a weight/volume measurement! Confused? Let me give you an example: If you reconstitute 600mg benzylpenicillin with 10ml water, you will make a solution strength of 600mg/10ml (see Figure 15).

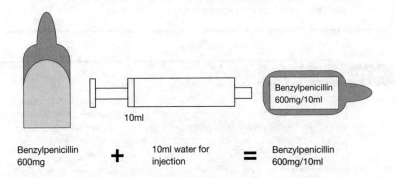

Benzylpenicillin
600mg

+

10ml water for
injection

=

Benzylpenicillin
600mg/10ml

Figure 15 Illustration of the reconstitution of 600mg benzypenicillin with 10ml water for injection

Warning!
If you are following this so far, I wonder whether you have considered what might be a problem with reconstituting drugs and how this could be avoided in practice? What could happen if I was in a hurry and feeling so pressured that I reconstituted the benzylpenicillin and drew up the 10ml really quickly, not noticing that there was still some of the benzylpenicillin powder at the bottom of the ampoule that hadn't dissolved? Would I be administering 600mg in my 10ml volume? It is really important to ensure that all the drug has dissolved into the liquid being added before the volume to be administered is drawn up. One of the errors in intravenous administration is nurses not leaving the drug to dissolve in the liquid for long enough and therefore administering the wrong dose to the patient (Wirtz et al., 2003).

Warning!
The other error which has been observed in practice is nurses reconsti-tuting the drug and preparing it ready for administration and then leaving it in the treatment room for a prolonged period of time before adminis-tering (Kopp et al., 2006). Remember that the drug is manufactured as a powder specifically because it is unstable in a liquid and loses its properties. Drawing it up and leaving it for extended time in the liquid form defeats the whole object of ensuring it is in a powder form so it doesn't lose its properties! Most importantly, though, it means that

when the nurse does administer the drug, it is likely to be less effective for the patient. It is recommended that reconstituted medication must be given within a specific time frame to ensure that the drug is still effective. You will need to refer to drug manufacturers' recommendations for each medication to find out the recommended time frame between reconstituting and administering the drug.

✳ Clinical Context

With most antibiotics it is common practice to draw up 10ml water for injection and inject only enough water into the ampoule to dissolve the drug. Once dissolved, the contents of the ampoule are drawn up into the 10ml syringe and shaken so that the drug is mixed into the 10ml. The reason for this is because antibiotics drugs are very strong. If the drug was dissolved in a small amount of water, this would give a very concentrated solution which can irritate and damage the veins when administered intravenously. Making a weaker solution through using 10ml to dissolve the drug reduces the irritation to the veins. Some antibiotics such as benzylpenicillin are so irritable to the veins that they must be further dissolved into a larger volume, usually an infusion bag, to make the solution weaker. Information about diluting volumes can be found in individual clinical areas.

EXERCISE 20

Consider the following drugs that are manufactured as a powder in an ampoule and, for each of the volumes indicated, write what is the new weight/volume strength that has been made.
1. 250mg ampoule of amoxicillin, 5ml of water for injection added.
2. 500mg flucloxacillin, 10ml water for injection added.
3. 600mg ampoule of benzylpenicillin, 10ml water for injection added.

(Answers: page 224)

Once you have worked out what weight/volume dosage you have now made, you can continue the calculation as you would for other weight/volume strength ampoules. However, generally in practice it is usual to look at the dosage prescribed and the dosage contained in the ampoule and consider the relationship between them to decide the volume of water for reconstituting.

For example, a prescription that is 150mg and an ampoule that is 200mg gives me the relationship of three-quarters or I could see that I can divide 200mg into four and then would need to administer three parts of these. Nurses can then decide the most appropriate volume to reconstitute the drug with to suit this calculation. For example, I may use 2ml and draw up 1.5ml or 4ml and draw up 3ml. Whatever volume I use, as long as I draw up three parts of the total drug dosage it will be 150mg.

✳ Clinical Context

The volume used depends on how you will be administering the drug. For example, if I was injecting the medication just under the subcutaneous layer of skin, that is, subcutaneously (SC), I would need a smaller volume. However, if I was to administer the drug into a large muscle, that is, intramuscularly (IM), then, as this is a larger area, I could administer a bigger volume. This knowledge will come with experience and familiarity with reconstituting drugs in practice.

EXERCISE 21

1. Your patient requires 500mg flucloxacillin. You reconstitute the 500mg ampoule with 10ml water for injections. How much of the 10ml do you need to administer?
2. Your patient requires 20mg of a drug. You reconstitute the 50mg drug ampoule with 5ml water. What volume of this do you need to administer?
3. You need to administer 125mg amoxicillin. The ampoules contain 250mg amoxicillin. You add 5ml to one ampoule and draw this up into a 5ml syringe. How much of this 5ml do you need to administer?
4. Your patient requires a subcutaneous injection of 10mg of a drug. The ampoules available are 20mg. How much water for injection would you add and how much would you administer (there is more than one answer).
5. You reconstitute 50mg of a drug with 2ml water. Your patient requires 40mg of this drug. How much would you administer?

(Answers: page 224)

● Chapter Summary

This chapter has explained medications where the strength is expressed as a weight and a volume and given a range of methods you can use to calculate doses using these medications. I have also built on the learning you did in Chapter 1 on dosages given according to a person's weight and we have applied these principles to weight/volume strength medications. Finally, I have explained how drugs can be reconstituted and some calculations involving this method. To see if you have understood what we have covered in this chapter, have a go at Assessment 2.

Assessment 2

Use the medicine chart and drug information below to complete the following exercise:

Sunnydene and Reynold NHS Trust

Name: Jerome Jackson   **Hospital Number:** 00124532

Weight: 45kg   **Height:** 152cm

REGULAR PRESCRIPTIONS

Year 2011		Date & Month 1st February		Date Time											
Drug Frusemide				07.00											
				09.00											
Dose 30mg	Route IV	Start date 1/2/11	Valid period 14 days	12.00											
				14.00											
Signature R Dickinson		Dispensed 1/2/11		18.00											
				22.00											
Additional comments															
Drug Morphine sulphate				07.00											
				09.00											
Dose 20mg	Route IM	Start date 1/2/11	Valid period 2 days	12.00											
				14.00											
Signature R Dickinson		Dispensed 1/2/11		18.00											
				22.00											
Additional comments															

Sunnydene and Reynold NHS Trust

Name: Akiko Oki   **Hospital Number:** 00056443

Weight: 32kg   **Height:** 134cm

REGULAR PRESCRIPTIONS

Year 2011		Date & Month 1st February		Date Time															
Drug **Amoxicillin**				07.00															
				09.00															
Dose 250mg	Route Po	Start date 1/2/11	Valid period 14 days	12.00															
				14.00															
Signature R Dickinson		Dispensed 1/2/11		18.00															
				22.00															
Additional comments																			
Drug **Paracetamol**				07.00															
				09.00															
Dose 0.25g	Route Po	Start date 1/2/11	Valid period 2 days	12.00															
				14.00															
Signature R Dickinson		Dispensed 1/2/11		18.00															
				22.00															
Additional comments No more than 4 doses in 24 hours (1g)																			

Sunnydene and Reynold NHS Trust

Name: Jane Simpson   **Hospital Number:** 02235343

Weight: 12.5kg   **Height:** 96cm

REGULAR PRESCRIPTIONS

Year 2011		Date & Month 1st February		Date Time																
Drug **Cefuroxime**				07.00																
				09.00																
Dose 30mg/kg	Route IM	Start date 1/2/11	Valid period 14 days	12.00																
				14.00																
Signature R Dickinson		Dispensed 1/2/11		18.00																
				22.00																
Additional comments																				

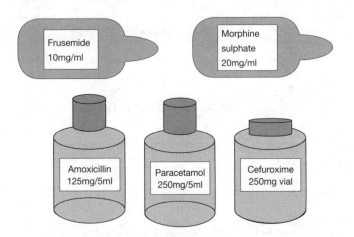

1. Calculate how many millilitres/ampoules of the available frusemide you would administer to Jerome Jackson.

2. How many millilitres/ampoules of the available morphine sulphate would you administer to Jerome Jackson?

3. How many millilitres of the available amoxicillin would you administer to Akiko Oki?

4. How many millilitres of the available paracetamol would you administer to Akiko Oki?

5. How many ampoules of the available cefuroxime would you administer to Jane Simpson?

6. Your patient has been prescribed 15mg of a drug that needs to be administered SC (subcutaneously). The available ampoules contain 20mg in powder form. If you reconstitute this with 2ml water for injection, how many millilitres do you need to administer your patient to give the 15mg dose?

7. Your patient has been prescribed 4mg/kg gentamicin IM (intramuscularly). Your patient weighs 45kg and the available ampoules contain 40mg/ml. How many millilitres do you need to administer?

8. You need to administer 0.6mg hyoscine hydrobromide IM to your patient. The ampoules available contain 400mcg/ml. How many millilitres/ampoules do you need to administer?

9. Your patient has been written up for 10mg/kg vancomycin IV (intravenously). Your patient weighs 15kg. The available vials are 250mg in powder form (that is, requires reconstitution). If you reconstitute the vial with 10ml water for injection, how any millilitres do you need to add to the infusion bag to give the required dosage?

10. Your patient has been prescribed benzylpenicillin 1.8g. The ampoules available contain 600mg in powder form. How many ampoules do you need to administer?

(Answers: page 224)

References

Kopp, B., Erstad, B., Allen, M., Theodorou, A. and Priestly, G. (2006) 'Medication errors an adverse drug events in an intensive care unit: direct observation approach for detection', *Critical Care Medicine* 34(2): 415–25.

Wirtz, V., Taxis, K. and Barber, N. (2003) 'An observational study of intravenous medication errors in the United Kingdom and in Germany', *Pharmacy World and Science* 25(3): 104–11.

Wright, K. (2008) 'Drug calculations part 1: a critique of the formula used by nurses', *Nursing Standard* 22(36): 40–3.

3 The Final Step! Calculations involving continuous infusions

Finishing touches and completing your understanding

This chapter explores:

▶ Calculations involving fluid replacement therapy
▶ Calculations using syringe pumps; dosages per hour and per patient weight
▶ Calculations involving syringe drivers

● **Infusions**

So far we have talked about drug dosages that involve both a weight and a volume measurement which are for the administration of medications as single dosages. These are known as bolus doses as the whole amount of the dosage is administered in one go. Pharmaceutically this means that the level of the drug will be at its peak when it is administered, but due to the drug's half-life (the time taken for the plasma concentration of the drug to halve), this will decrease until the next dose.

Ideally, the dosages are sufficiently spaced out throughout the day so that a therapeutic level of the drug remains in the patient's body. This is the reason why it is important that dosages are not missed and are given as close to the prescribed time as possible. It is important that the principle of bolus dosages is considered when managing patient absences from the ward or other reasons for missed dosages.

In order to ensure a more exact and stable level of a drug in a patient's system, drugs can be given continuously (see Figure 16). Drugs given continuously are usually given as infusions. These infusions can be administered subcutaneously, but most often intravenously. There are various devices available to administer continuous infusions of drugs. These include electronic infusion devices such as volumetric infusion pumps, syringe pumps and syringe drivers and manual giving sets (see Box 14).

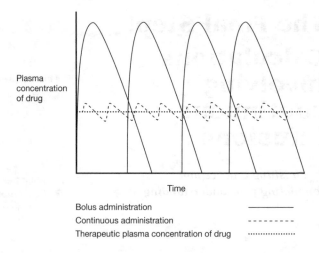

Figure 16 Diagram showing difference in plasma concentration levels between bolus and continuously infused drugs

Box 14 Different types of electronic devices for infusions

Electronic devices have two methods of functioning. The volumetric infusion device involves the fluid being moved along the tubing by a peristalsis-like action as the tubing is compressed and released by a set of rollers or protrusions. Syringe pumps and syringe drivers have a motor that activates a screw and gradually compresses the plunger on a syringe.

There are various makes of electronic pumps available, each with different programming requirements and you need to refer to the manufacturers' instructions for use. Most pumps come with built-in safety functions that prevent tampering and indicate when the infusion is not running as programmed, for example due to an occlusion (an obstruction or closure).

Some electronic pumps are designed to be attached to a standard infusion drip stand, allowing them to be moved easily. There are many new pumps available that are smaller and designed to be portable for patient comfort and independence. These usually come with carrying pouches, for example chemotherapy pumps and syringe drivers.

- **Volumetric infusion pumps** – used for infusing large volumes such as fluid replacement or specific pumps for administering parenteral nutrition (intravenous feeding)
- **Syringe pumps** – used for small volumes of medication that need to be administered continuously, for example insulin
- **Syringe drivers** – used for administering medication subcutaneously
- **Patient controlled analgesia (PCA)** – similar to a syringe pump, but specifically designed to administer a set amount of medication when activated by a hand-held device controlled by the patient. A PCA device has additional built-in safety functions that prevent multiple doses being administered in specific time periods

Although the electronic devices assist with ensuring a continuous amount of drug is administered to the patient, they can't do this unless they are programmed correctly to administer the prescribed amount and the correct dosage is placed into the device. So there is no getting away from understanding calculations and solving them even with electronic devices!

Once again, the important thing for setting up infusions is understanding what it is you are trying to do. Once this is clear, it is easier to set out the calculation and work out what is required to programme the electronic devices.

Warning!
You should never use an electronic device without receiving appropriate training first.

The general principle of continuous infusions is that a small amount of the drug or fluid is given to the patient continuously throughout the infusion time. For fluid replacement, this is the difference between gulping a large glass of water every 4 hours for a 12-hour period and sipping the water throughout the 12 hours.

Before volumetric pumps were used, infusions would be given manually using giving sets. This method is not always consistent as the infusion speed can be altered by many different factors including the position of the infusion bag and the patient's arm. To ensure that there was some control of infusions a burette would have been used.

Burettes consist of a chamber above the drip dial into which a set amount of fluid from the infusion bag can be decanted. Once this chamber is empty, no more fluid will be administered until the chamber is refilled (see Figure 17). This way nurses can have more control over how much of the infusion a patient is administered for a set time.

Nowadays, instead of the chamber and the giving set being used to control the amount administered over an hour, most clinical areas have volumetric pumps, which regulate the amount of drug the patient is administered, drip by drip, allowing a much finer control over the continuousness of the infusion.

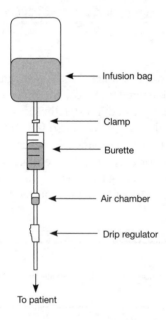

Figure 17 Illustration of a burette in practice

● Fluid Replacement Therapy

Although I have talked about manual giving sets and burettes as if these were last used by Ms Nightingale herself, in actual fact in some areas they are still used. Volumetric infusion pumps, although more accurate and safer, are not always available due to resource constraints and so infusions where the accuracy of the administration is not vital may still be administered using a manual giving set.

To understand how to calculate infusion rates I always think it's helpful to first understand what it is exactly you are trying to do. Fluid replacement therapy may be prescribed for a variety of reasons but is generally necessary when the patient is unable to take the required fluids orally for whatever reason. Fluid replacement therapy is nearly always given intravenously. On occasions, fluids may be administered subcutaneously, but this is more for palliative reasons and is rarely used.

Patients will be prescribed a set amount of a specific fluid to be administered over a set amount of time. For example, a patient may be prescribed 1000ml of 0.9% sodium chloride over 10 hours. The aim of the infusion is to ensure an equal amount of the 1000ml 0.9% sodium chloride is administered throughout the 10 hours. It is no good the patient receiving 200ml for the first hour, then nothing for 6 hours then 800ml in the final 3 hours of the infusion. An equal amount needs to be administered over the whole 10 hours.

Let's consider the hourly rate first. The patient requires 1000ml divided in equal amounts to be administered every hour for a total of 10 hours. This is similar to the divided dosages calculations you did in Chapter 1. You are dividing the total volume required by the number of hours this needs to be administered over. In this example the answer would be 100ml to be administered every hour. If this isn't totally clear don't worry, but have a look at Figure 18 below.

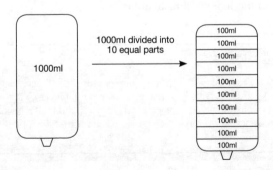

Figure 18 An illustration of rate per hour for a 1000ml infusion bag
prescribed over 10 hours

For this infusion, the amount infused every hour would be 100ml. Ten lots of 100ml would give a total of 1000ml infused over 10 hours. The volume per hour of infusions is known as the rate per hour or hourly rate. So for the example above the rate per hour would be written as 100ml/hour (100ml/hr). The calculation you are doing to work out the hourly rate for fluid replacement infusions is:

$$\frac{\text{volume to be infused (ml)}}{\text{infusion time (hours)}} = \text{rate per hour}$$

> **? Maths Explained**
>
> In order to solve rate-per-hour questions without a calculator, you will need to ensure that you are confident with using long division or learn the frequent patterns that occur commonly in infusion rate calculations (see tips for learning below).

Volumetric Infusion Devices

There are some volumetric pumps that are extremely helpful and clever. These devices only require you to programme in the volume to be infused and the infusion time and it will do everything else for you. Other devices want you to do a little bit of work and need the rate per hour programmed in. For all infusions, though, you will need to be familiar with obtaining the information from the infusion charts and programming the specific infusion devices found in your clinical areas.

> **✔ Tips for Learning**
>
> Once you have worked out the rate per hour, do the calculation again backwards to make sure that this volume multiplied by the number of hours the infusion is running at will give you the total infusion volume. So, using the example above, I would check that ten lots of 100ml will give the total 1000ml.

To check you are happy with rate-per-hour calculations, I have given you some questions to answer in Exercise 22:

EXERCISE 22

1. A patient requires 1000ml 5% glucose to run over 8 hours. What is the rate per hour required?
2. A patient is prescribed 500ml 0.9% sodium chloride over 8 hours. Calculate the hourly rate for this infusion.
3. Your patient has been prescribed 1000ml dextrose saline over 12 hours. What is the hourly infusion rate?
4. You need to infuse your patient with 500ml Hartmann's over 4 hours. What rate per hour would you set up an infusion pump for?
5. An infusion of 500ml 5% glucose is prescribed over 6 hours. What is the hourly rate for this infusion?

(Answers: page 226)

✔ **Tips for Learning**

Generally, the mathematical principle for rounding numbers applies for the rate per hour. Numbers are rounded to the nearest whole number. Numbers which are 5 or above are rounded up and those which are 4 and below are rounded down. For example, 83.3ml/hr would be rounded down to 83ml/hr and 21.7ml/hr would be rounded up to 22ml/hr.

✔ **Tips for Learning**

You may have already noticed a pattern with the answers to the exercise above. The infusion amounts prescribed and the duration of infusions are often repeated so it is possible to become familiar with these and know immediately the rate per hour without doing any calculation. The common infusion calculations for rate per hour are:

1000ml over 12 hours = 83ml/hr
1000ml over 10 hours = 100ml/hr
1000ml over 8 hours = 125ml/hr
 500ml over 4 hours = 125ml/hr
 500ml over 6 hours = 83ml/hr
 500ml over 8 hours = 63ml/hr

You may also see that 1000ml over 12 hours is the same as 500ml over 6 hours and 1000ml over 8 hours is the same as 500ml over 4 hours. These patterns are helpful so in time you will be able to calculate automatically the infusion rate per hour and won't need to carry out cumbersome long division.

Initially, though, it is always better to actually do the calculation so you are sure and begin to learn these patterns. Some nurses carry the common infusion rates around with them so that they can refer to them rather than calculate it fresh each time. I would personally recommend learning these infusion rates but always checking that you are correct before administering either through calculating or referring to your own notes.

Manual Infusions

So far I have explained how to calculate the infusion rate a patient requires per hour. Setting the infusion to run through an electronic device will ensure that the volume being infused every hour is divided equally between every minute and second so that a continuous amount is given over that hour and every hour. If you do not have an electronic device to do this for you, then you will need to use a manual giving set to set the flow of the infusion so that it runs equally over the infusion time.

Let's start where we left off having calculated the rate per hour. Imagine that you were gleefully about to programme the rate per hour into your electronic device when ICU (intensive care unit) ring and say they need the pump urgently. As you watch your electronic pump being whisked away out of the ward, you realise that you will have to use the manual giving set which requires you to calculate the volume per minute.

The volume you were about to programme in was 100ml per hour for 10 hours. Now you could just set your mobile alarm (not that you would have this available during duty of course!) and go to the patient every hour and infuse roughly 100ml for the next 10 hours, but, as has already been mentioned, this wouldn't ensure a continuous amount of fluid. We know that the patient requires 100ml every hour. What would the rate per minute be for this infusion? How many millilitres would need to be infused every minute so that 100ml is infused in total over one hour? This calculation follows the same principle as the one you did before to work out the rate per hour; you would divide the volume to be infused by the duration:

$$\frac{\text{volume to be infused}}{\text{duration in hours}} = \text{rate per hour} \qquad \frac{\text{rate per hour}}{60} = \text{rate per minute}$$

$$\frac{1000}{10} = 100\text{ml} \qquad\qquad \frac{100}{60} = 1.66\text{ml}$$

The rate per minute can be rounded up to 1.7ml. Now you may be thinking how ridiculous this is getting as there is no way you could infuse 1.7ml per minute as it's such a tiny amount. And you would be right, it would be hard on your own to do this but you have the underrated clever little giving set to help you.

Now giving sets work by having a tube that attaches to the infusion bag. When the bag is positioned so that it is higher than the patient, the fluid runs down the tube as a result of gravity. The higher the infusion bag, the quicker the fluid will run. The fluid from the infusion drips into a chamber that is half filled with the fluid to prevent air bubbles and then flows into the infusion line. This is the same as the infusion representation in Figure 17 but without the burette.

The clever part of giving sets is that they are manufactured so that they produce a consistent drop size and allow the number of drips that are needed to make 1ml to be known. For example, most giving sets are manufactured so that 20 drips will give 1ml fluid. Using this principle you can then work out that 10 drops would give 0.5ml fluid and 40 drops would give 2ml fluid. The number of drops that give 1ml of fluid is written on the back of the giving set packet and is called the drop factor (see Figure 19).

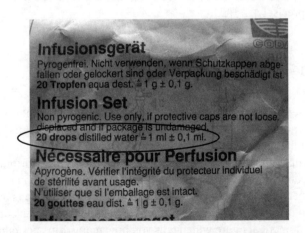

Figure 19 A giving set packet showing the number of drops/ml

In order to regulate the flow of fluid, giving sets have a regulator that consists of a plastic device which makes the lumen of the infusion tube smaller so less fluid can get through. This slows the rate of the drops. The drop size remains the same but the rate at which the drops are infused is less.

Now if you are still with me, let's go back to you on the ward with your infusion all ready to go, your new-found respect for the humble giving set and your calculation to date which is 1.7ml per minute. Now if you know that 20 drops of this giving set give 1ml, and you set up the infusion so that it allows 20 drops per minute, the patient would be infused 1ml every minute.

This is less than you need as you want 1.7ml per minute. To work out how many drips would give 1.7ml, you need to multiply this by 20. This is 34 drops.

> ✔ **Tips for Learning**
>
> You can do a calculation such as 1.7 × 20 by calculating 1.7 × 10 twice. This is 17 + 17 which gives 34.

Now every minute the patient will receive 34 drops, which is 1.7ml. Every hour, this would add up to be 60 lots of 1.7, which is 102ml, and over 10 hours this would be 1020ml (don't worry that it is not 1000ml exactly; with giving sets it is often an approximation. This is one of the reasons that volumetric pumps are so imperative for patients who need their infusion regulated precisely).

34 drops   = 1.7ml
60 lots of 1.7ml = 102ml
10 lots of 100ml = 1020ml

Please do not worry if your eyes have glazed over and you haven't followed me. I really just want you to understand the principle of using a giving set and to learn to give them a little credit for the amazing job they do! Thankfully, the long-winded procedure I've explained to work out the rate to set up a manual giving set has been simplified into a formula.

This means, luckily for those who haven't followed this completely, that you don't need to worry too much. All you do with the formula is put in the corresponding numerical figures from practice and solve the calculation to arrive at a numerical figure which tells you how many drips per minute you need to set the infusion for it to give the right volume.

Formula

$$\frac{\text{volume to be infused (ml)}}{\text{duration (hours)}} \times \frac{\text{drop factor}}{60} = \text{drips per minute (dpm)}$$

The procedure I've gone through basically explains the formula. Often, student nurses in particular can set up the formula and solve the calculation, but don't understand what the number that they've arrived at means and what they need to do with this.

✔ **Tips for Learning**

To make sure that your answer is right you need to be thinking logically and considering what a reasonable answer would be from your clinical experience. Answers such as 3 drips per minute or 340 drips per minute should set alarm bells ringing – even if not straight away, I hope that they will be ringing very loudly once you try to regulate the giving set to these rates!

The formula gives you the number of drips you need to regulate the giving set to over one minute. Once you have calculated the number of drips the giving set needs to be set at over a minute, you then need to adjust the regulator on the giving set and count the number of drips until you have adjusted it sufficiently to give approximately that number of drips over the minute. As you become more experienced, you will begin to be able to judge the speed required for the drips per minute required.

Those of you that are very observant will perhaps notice that the first part of the formula gives you the rate per hour. The second part uses the knowledge of the drop factor of the giving set (remember, this is the number of drops which will give you 1ml) and uses 60 to convert the rate into minutes.

Warning!
You may be thinking: what is the point of calculating the drip per minute precisely if you then have to adjust it throughout according to the amount of infusion going through? You have got a valid point and some nurses don't actually calculate the drips per minute at all but just estimate the speed and come back and vary this throughout. I would always advise that you calculate the actual drip rate for two reasons:
1. To help you become familiar with this calculation and understand exactly what it is you are doing
2. For professional and legal reasons.
If there is a problem with an infusion, for example it went through far too quickly and caused the patient harm, when questioned you need to be able to say the rate that you set the infusion up at. This demonstrates your professionalism and evidences that you understand infusions and how to work out and set the rate. Telling a court of law that you guessed the rate from your experience will probably not help your case!

Here is an example to see how the formula works and perhaps judge which way you find easier: using the formula or my long-winded procedure! To make it fair we should use the same example. So imagine your patient has been prescribed 1000ml 0.9% sodium chloride over 10 hours and the giving set has a drop factor of 20. The volume to be infused is 1000ml and the duration is 10 hours:

$$\frac{1000}{10} \times \frac{20}{60} = \text{drips per minute}$$

Now you can solve this calculation several ways:

● **Calculator** – If you are using a calculator you can do this by keying in the calculation using either of the two options here. Both options will give you the correct answer.

Option 1

1 0 0 0 × 2 0 ÷ 1 0 ÷ 6 0 =

Option 2

1 0 0 0 ÷ 1 0 × 2 0 ÷ 6 0 =

Warning!
A common mistake that nurses make is not keying in the numbers correctly and missing out a zero or adding a zero. This will make the answer ten times less or ten times more than it should be. Translating this to practice, it means the patient's infusion rate will be ten times faster or ten times slower than it should be. This can obviously have significant effects on the patient's health, depending on their condition.

● **Without a calculator** – Again there are different ways of solving this calculation manually. Firstly you can just use the numbers as they appear here and work out the solution to each part of the formula. So you could work out:

$$\frac{1000 \times 20}{10 \times 60} = \frac{20\,000}{600} = \frac{200}{6} = \frac{100}{3}$$

Many people are then familiar with reducing this fraction by cancelling the zeros from the 20 000 and 6000. The result, 200 divided by 6, can be further reduced by dividing top and bottom by 2 and 100 divided by 3 can worked out using long division:

$$
\begin{array}{r}
0\ \ 3\ \ 3\ .\ 3'^* \\
3\ \overline{)1\ _{1}0\ _{1}0\ .\ _{1}0}
\end{array}
$$

*see maths explained below

It is important you understand what it is that you are calculating so you can make sense of the numerical answer of 33.3 that your solution has given you. Remember, you are calculating how many drops you need to set the manual giving set for to ensure that a continuous and even amount of fluid is given. Your answer of 33.3 is the number of drops per minute.

We have talked about the necessity of rounding a number up or down to the nearest whole number before. We need to do this again here. You may be standing staring at the giving set for rather a long time trying to ensure that you set the regulator so that it gives 33 and a third of a drop per minute (n.b. 0.3 is approximately one-third). The giving set can only give whole drops and you cannot set it so that it gives you a part of a drop! So you have to round the number to the nearest whole number. In this example we would round the number down to give 33 drops per minute.

Warning!
Once you have set the manual giving set to the calculated number of drops per minute, it is vital that you go back regularly throughout the infusion duration to check that it is running correctly. As has been mentioned before, the position of the patient can alter the speed of the infusion and you must continue regulating the speed throughout the infusion. You can also do this by roughly checking that for a 10-hour infusion you would expect approximately a quarter of the infusion bag to have been used after 2.5 hours, half after 5 hours and so on. You can adjust the regulator accordingly if the infusion is not currently running to time.

? Maths Explained

Some answers that you work out using long division will continue to repeat themselves. You could continue to do the division or you can accept that the number will continue on and on (in fact it will continue for infinity!). When you have the same number repeating, rather than write out the same numbers until your arm aches or you run out of room, there is a mathematical convention which uses the apostrophe sign to mean that the number is recurring. So, as in the long division above, you may see 33.3' – this means that it is 33.3333333333333333 3333333333333333333333333333 for infinity!

✔ **Tips for Learning**

An easier way to solve the calculation would be to make the numbers in the calculation smaller using knowledge of equivalent fractions. Smaller numbers are easier to deal with. Also, large numbers of zeros are risky because it is so easy to miss one out. Reducing the numbers down requires knowledge of fractions and reducing fractions. If you are not confident doing this then you may wish to refresh these skills in Chapter 4.

? **Maths Explained**

To reduce the numbers in a calculation involving multiplication of fractions, you need to remember that you must reduce the number by the same amount in the top and bottom of the fraction (numerator and denominator). You can reduce the fractions between the top and bottom in one fraction and diagonally across the fractions. You **cannot** reduce fractions by dividing horizontally, that is, both the top numbers (numerator) or the bottom number (denominator).

$$\frac{1000}{10} \times \frac{20}{60}$$

So for the example here we can reduce the fractions by dividing by 10 to end up with:

$$\frac{100}{1} \times \frac{2}{6}$$

and then divide by 2 to be left with the calculation $100 \times 1/3 = 33.3'$

In clinical practice, to set up the formula and calculate the infusion rate you would look at the intravenous fluid medicine chart. Although there are variations in the chart layout according to the clinical area you are working in, generally it will consist of a table that provides you with the date to be infused, name of infusion, volume to be infused, duration for the infusion in hours, and the prescriber's signature (see example chart, Figure 20). To extract the information from this chart you would look along the columns and take out the relevant details and place these into the formula; for example volume to be infused and duration in hours. The drop factor details need to be extracted from the giving set packet you are planning to use to set the infusion up (see Figure 19).

Sunnydene and Reynold NHS Trust

Intravenous medicine administration chart

Name: Fred Kumar   **Hospital Number:** 0789655   **Consultant:** Rogers

Date of Birth: 1/9/1952   **Ward:** Oak

Date prescribed	Solution	Volume	Duration of Infusion	Date to be given	Prescriber's signature
1/2/2011	0.9% sodium chloride	1 Litre	10 hours	1/2/2011	R Dickenson

Figure 20 Intravenous medicine administration chart

When you are being asked to calculate a drip rate or rate per hour in a written test, this information is presented in a different form and you need to learn to extract the relevant information from the written question. Some students and nurses find this more difficult to do and become confused by the numbers used to identify the strength of particular infusions, for example 5% glucose and 0.9% sodium chloride.

I once had a student nurse tell me rather gleefully that my attempt at putting these numbers in to confuse them hadn't worked! Other students have also become baffled by these additional numbers and I have seen them make appearances in the formula calculation that they are trying to solve.

It is important in written questions that you read this carefully and try to imagine that you are in clinical practice to help you make sense of them. This will help you to extract the correct information. You also need to become familiar with the way that these written questions are expressed and the language used. I have given a common question for infusion rates below. I have translated the language used and highlighted the information that you need for the formula:

Question

Your patient has been prescribed **1000ml** 5% glucose over **10 hours**. The giving set drop factor is **20**. What rate would you set this infusion up for?

Translation

Your patient has been prescribed **1000ml** 5% glucose over **10 hours** – *A patient has been prescribed an infusion of 5% glucose. The volume of this infusion is 1000ml and the duration of the infusion required is 10 hours.*

The giving set drop factor is **20** – *On the back of the giving set packet the drop factor stated is 20 drops/ml.*

What rate would you set this infusion up for? – *How many drips per minute would you set the giving set up for?*

Now it is probably time for you to do some calculations yourself so you can experience what I am talking about. To summarise and to help you work your way logically through the questions, I have given a step-by-step guide to help you. I would suggest that you follow this guide initially until you become more confident and competent in calculating continuous infusion rates. Remember that you need to be as sufficiently confident in your answer to these questions here as you would be in clinical practice.

(a) Make sure you understand the question and what it is you are required to calculate

(b) Write down the formula and ensure this is correct

(c) Extract the relevant numbers from practice and place them into the formula

(d) Chose the method you wish to use, that is, calculator or arithmetically

(e) Solve the calculation

(f) Round your number to the nearest whole number

(g) Check your answer using a different method or repeating your calculation until you have a consistent numerical answer

(h) Using your knowledge of what it is you are trying to calculate, place your numerical solution back into context, for example rate per hour or drips per minute

(i) Check that the answer you have obtained makes sense logically and using your clinical practice experience

(j) Set the manual giving set to the required drip rate per minute (that is, number of drips) and volumetric device rate per hour (that is, number of millilitres per hour)

EXERCISE 23

1. Your patient has been prescribed 1000ml 0.9% sodium chloride infusion over 10 hours. The manual giving set drop factor is 20. Calculate the number of drops per minute you would set this infusion for.

2. You need to administer 500ml 5% glucose to your patient over 6 hours. The manual giving set has a drop factor of 20. What rate would you set this infusion up for?

3. Your patient requires a 500ml blood transfusion over 4 hours. The blood giving set has a drop factor of 15. How many drops per minute would you set this infusion up for?

4. You have been asked to set up an infusion of 1000ml dextrose saline over 8 hours. The manual giving set available has a drop factor of 20. How many drops per minute would you set this infusion for?

5. Your patient has been prescribed 1000ml 0.9% sodium chloride over 12 hours. If the giving set has a drop factor of 20, what rate would you set this infusion for?

(Answers: page 226)

✔ Tips for Learning

Once you become confident at calculating drip rates using the formula method you may notice a pattern emerging with the second part of the formula. Most giving sets have a drop factor of either 20 or 15. As the 60 for the minutes never changes in the formula, the second part of the calculation is often $^{20}/_{60}$ or $^{15}/_{60}$. You may notice that this can be reduced to $^{1}/_{3}$ or $^{1}/_{4}$. So a short cut for calculating the drip rate that I often use is the rate per hour divided by either 3 or 4, that is, a third or quarter of this. For the example above, it would be 100ml divided by 3, which I know is 33.3'.

✔ Tips for Learning

You can estimate the speed of the drops by comparing the number of drops per minute to the number of seconds, which is 60. For example, a rate of 34 drops per minute can be approximated to 30 drops per minute. Comparing 30 with the number of seconds of 60, you can work out the rate will be approximately 1 drop for every two seconds. This can help you to estimate the speed of the drops. This is illustrated in Box 15.

Box 15 Illustration of the drip rate compared to seconds

Drip rate	Seconds												Description
	1	2	3	4	5	6	7	8	9	10	11	12	
60	•	•	•	•	•	•	•	•	•	•	•	•	One drip per second
30	•		•		•		•		•		•		One drip every two seconds
40	•	•	•	•	•	•	•		•				Two drips every three seconds
20	•			•			•			•			One drip every three seconds

✔ Tips for Learning

Remember, a previous tip for working out rates per hour was to learn the rates per hour for the common prescriptions of volumes and durations of infusions. You can also do this for the drip rate. Many nurses used to carry these drip rates around with them, usually carefully written on a wooden tongue depressor kept in their pocket! Now with the introduction and common usage of volumetric pumps this isn't so necessary. However, you will still have to calculate drip rates from time to time and therefore you need to keep these skills up. It is better therefore to calculate each drip rate using the formula rather than using an aide memoir, although these can be useful as a checking aid and for learning the common drip rates in practice so you can easily spot any errors you've made in your calculation. You might like to photocopy Box 16, which gives the common rates for continuous intravenous infusions.

Box 16 Common rates for continuous intravenous infusions

Volume (ml) and duration (hr)	Rate per hour	Drips per minute (Drop factor 20)	Drips per minute (Drop factor 15)
1000ml over 12 hours	83	28	
1000ml over 10 hours	100	33	
1000ml over 8 hours	125	42	
500ml over 8 hours	63	21	
500ml over 6 hours	83		21
500ml over 4 hours	125		31

EXERCISE 24

1. Your patient has been prescribed 1000ml 0.9% sodium chloride over 8 hours. Using a manual giving set with a drop factor of 20 drops/ml, calculate the number of drops per minute you would set this infusion rate for.

2. Your patient has been written up for a 1000ml infusion of 5% dextrose over 12 hours. What rate per hour would you set this infusion for using a volumetric pump?

3. You need to set up a unit of blood (500ml) for your patient to run over 2 hours. The giving set has a drop factor of 15 drops/ml. How many drips per minute would you set this infusion for?

4. The next IV infusion your patient has been written up for is now due and is 500ml dextrose saline over 6 hours. What rate per hour would you set for this infusion using a volumetric pump?

5. Your colleague has set up a 1000ml infusion of 5% dextrose prescribed to run over 10 hours at a rate of 125ml/hr. The infusion was commenced at 8am. What time would this infusion finish? Was this the correct rate?

(Answers: page 227)

Percentages

We have already seen that the strength of fluid replacement infusions is given in percentages. So, for example, you may see glucose infusions which are different strengths, that is, 5% or 10% glucose. The percentages tell you the strength of the glucose or sodium chloride that the infusion contains. You can probably work out easily that the 10% glucose infusion bag would contain more glucose than a similar volume of 5% glucose.

The infusions have been manufactured by dissolving the required crystal in water. For each infusion strength, a different amount of the solid has been dissolved in the fluid. This is the same as dissolving sugar in your tea. The more teaspoons of sugar you dissolve in it, then the stronger the taste of sugar in your tea.

✳ Clinical Context

A crystalloid is an infusion that contains 'salts' which have been dissolved into a liquid. Once a solid has been dissolved it is known as a solute. When the infusion is heated and the liquid has evaporated, the 'salts' are left as a crystal at the bottom, hence their name. Other infusions are called colloids because the solid added does not dissolve into the liquid but remains suspended within it, for example gelofusine and Hartmann's. The difference clinically is that crystalloids can diffuse across cell membranes and colloids cannot. This means that crystalloids are used to increase the amount of fluid available in the body and colloids are used to increase the volume of blood.

In practice, generally, you are only required to understand the concept of percentages and know that a 10% infusion bag of glucose is stronger than a 5% infusion bag. However, in written tests you may be asked to calculate the weight of a solute that a particular infusion bag contains.

Although this calculation is not required in practice, it is useful to understand exactly how much of a particular solute an infusion bag contains so you can understand clinically what you are administering to your patient.

I once worked with a nurse who set up an infusion of 5% glucose for a patient who was diabetic, with blood sugars controlled with insulin. The nurse set the infusion up *correctly* using a manual giving set to run over 8 hours. When the nurse came back to check the infusion an hour later, however, *the patient had moved the position of their arm so that the infusion had speeded up* and the whole amount had gone through! What do you think happened to the patient's blood sugars? Why had this happened? The answer to this if you are unsure will become clear as we practise calculating how much each infusion bag contains of the solute.

Let's go back to the manufacturing stage of the infusions. The chemists in their white coats are there with their giant pots of water. Into the first pot they add glucose, into the second pot some sodium chloride and finally to the third pot they add both glucose and sodium chloride. They gather round their pots and stir slowly until the solids have dissolved and they're left with just liquid.

Once all the solid has dissolved, they pour the liquids into the waiting infusion bags which can contain 1000ml and 500ml. Finally, they need to label the bags to show what strength of solute is in each bag. To work out the strength, the chemists need to know how much volume they started with and how much weight of the solid they added. This is similar to the principle of how ampoules are made.

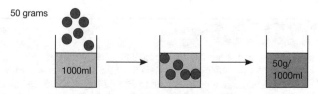

Figure 21 Illustration of how a 5% infusion is 'made'

However, the difference with infusions is that, instead of expressing what amount of weight per volume is in each ampoule, the strength is expressed as a percentage. This means that you need to understand the principle of percentages.

A percentage basically means per hundred (cent means one hundred, for example 100 cents in one dollar and a century means one hundred years). So infusion strengths are expressed as how many grams of the salt have been dissolved in one hundred millilitres of fluid. In Figure 21 the chemists have made a solution containing:

50 grams in 1000mls

Remember the principle of the marriage between volume and weight, that they are forever entwined and you cannot do something to one without the same thing happening to the other? If therefore I want to know the percentage, I need to know how many grams are in 100ml. To do this I would need one-tenth of 1000ml and therefore I would have one-tenth of 50 grams. Mathematically, this means I divide both the 50g and 1000ml by 10 to get:

5g in 100ml, which is 5%

> **? Maths Explained**
>
> You can work the percentage out using a set calculation if this makes you feel more secure. This is:
>
> $$\frac{50}{1000} \times 100 = 5\%$$

I now have the number of grams expressed out of one hundred, which is the percentage strength. Therefore a 1000ml 5% glucose infusion bag would contain 50g.

Going back to the example of the nurse on a ward who had realised that 1000ml 5% glucose had been infused to their patient in one hour. How many grams of glucose had they just given this poor patient? Hopefully you worked out that they'd given 50g glucose! Bearing in mind that one teaspoon of sugar is approximately equivalent to 5g, they had in effect given the patient 10 teaspoons of sugar over one hour. It is of little surprise then that the patient's blood sugar was elevated.

> ✳ **Clinical Context**
>
> The infusion 0.9% sodium chloride is often also called normal saline. Officially, normal saline could be any infusion containing sodium chloride of varying strength, which is why some people insist that the correct name and strength is always used.

I know I have explained this in great detail and perhaps laboriously, but as I have repeatedly said, you need to understand what it is you are calculating first so you can make sense of the maths and visualise clinically what it is you are doing.

I hope that the explanation has helped you to understand how infusion strengths are manufactured and worked out. And now that I have apologised for my long explanation, you'll perhaps forgive me for going back to the laboratory where the chemists in white coats have finished labelling the glucose bag as 5% strength but need some help with the sodium chloride and glucose and sodium chloride mixtures.

Pot 2 – the chemists dissolved 9 grams sodium chloride into 1000ml water:

9g in 1000ml
0.9g in 100ml

Therefore the solution strength made is 0.9% sodium chloride.

Pot 3 – the chemists dissolved 1.8g sodium chloride and 40 grams glucose into 1000ml water:

1.8g in 1000ml sodium chloride
0.18g in 100ml
40g in 1000ml glucose
4g in 100ml

Therefore the solution strength made is 0.18% sodium chloride and 4% glucose (also known as dextrose saline).

Now we have done the calculation back to front so far, by working out what the strength of solution would be, given that amount of solid and volume. Generally in clinical practice and in written assessments, the question will start with the percentage strength of an infusion bag and ask how many grams of the solute the bag contains. For example, a question may be:

How many grams of glucose are there in a 1000ml 5% glucose infusion bag?

For these questions you need to remember what we have previously shown, which is that the percentage means how many grams of solid have been dissolved in 100ml fluid. So, for the example above, we know that 5% means that the solution contains 5g in every 100ml so, to find out how many grams are in 1000ml, we need to multiply these amounts by 10:

5g in 100ml
50g in 1000ml

The answer then is 1000ml 5% glucose contains 50g glucose.

EXERCISE 25

1. How many grams of glucose are in a 1000ml 10% glucose infusion bag?
2. How many grams of sodium chloride are in a 500ml 0.9% sodium chloride infusion bag?
3. How many grams of glucose are in a 500ml 5% glucose infusion bag?

(Answers: page 227)

In the answers for Exercise 25 (see page 227), I have deliberately explained how to work out these questions using the above methods, as I believe that they help you to keep in mind what it is you are trying to work out and involve a simple manipulation of numbers.

Some of you may remember being taught a different method to calculate percentages. This method uses the same principle that a percentage is an amount out of one hundred and thus can be expressed as a fraction. Once you have completed the calculation, you need to relate it back to the question to find out what the numerical answer actually means. For example, 5 out of a potential 100 can be expressed as:

$$\frac{5}{100}$$

To work out 5% of a number therefore involves the percentage fraction of the number, which would be:

$$\frac{5}{100} \times \text{number}$$

For the infusion questions, 5% glucose would be:

$$\frac{5}{100} \times 1000ml = \frac{5000}{100} = 50 \qquad \text{putting this back into context} = 50g$$

Therefore a useful formula would be:

$$\frac{\text{percentage of solute}}{100} \times \text{volume of infusion} = \text{grams of solute}$$

Use this method for Exercise 26.

EXERCISE 26

1. How many grams of glucose in a 10% 500ml infusion bag?
2. How many grams of 0.9% sodium chloride in a 1000ml infusion bag?
3. How many grams of glucose in a 500ml 4% dextrose saline infusion bag?

(Answers: page 228)

Whenever you come across percentages now, hopefully you will be able to remember that it always means out of one hundred, and for infusion bags, it is always the number of grams out of the 100ml volume. If you are having difficulty with understanding this, please don't worry. Percentages are explained in more detail in Chapter 4 of this book, so you can work through this and then come back to it when you are feeling more confident.

● Syringe Pumps

We have gone through fluid replacement infusions, so far, looking at calculations involving rate per hour for using volumetric pumps and drips per minute for manual giving sets. Other continuous infusions that are given in clinical practice and involve calculations are intravenous infusions which contain medication.

Continuous infusions of medication require different calculations and administration, depending on the clinical need of the patient. Some infusions, for example heparin, can be prescribed as a set amount which needs to be administered over 24 hours. Other patients may need this heparin administered continuously as a set amount per hour. We will go through each of the different calculations in this section.

Warning!
Sometimes the term syringe pump can be used synonymously with syringe driver. The name for the electronic device often depends on the clinical area you are working in. In the community, a syringe driver is a device that is used to administer, usually morphine, over a 12-hour or 24-hour period and is not the same as a syringe driver used on an acute ward. To save confusion, I always refer to the electronic device for the ward as a syringe pump and the syringe driver as the device mainly used for palliative care.

Syringe pumps over 24 hours

Some medications are prescribed as a dosage to be administered over a 24-hour period. For example, a patient may be prescribed 25 000 units of heparin over 24 hours. Continuous infusions of medications are administered using a syringe pump. A syringe pump is so called because it works by slowly depressing a syringe to administer the infusion. The syringe pump is programmed to depress the syringe a set number of millilitres per hour. Like the volumetric pumps for administrating infusions, the syringe administers the millilitres of fluid gradually and steadily over each hour.

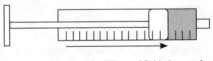

Number of millilitres of fluid given so far

Figure 22 A syringe showing rate of millilitres/hr

Now if I filled a syringe with water, put it in the syringe pump and set the rate for 1ml to be administered every hour for 24 hours, how many millilitres would be administered in total? If one millilitre is administered per hour, then over 24 hours this would be 24ml.

✱ Clinical Context

The syringe is attached to an infusion line which then attaches to the patient's intravenous access point, for example peripheral cannula. To set up the syringe pump, the syringe needs to be filled with the required volume and then the infusion line needs to be 'primed', that is, filled with the fluid, like an intravenous giving set, to prevent an air embolus entering the veins. The volume required to prime the infusion line is 2ml.

We have worked out that if I set the pump to administer 1ml per hour, it would administer 24ml over 24 hours. If I set the pump to administer 2ml per hour, it would administer 48ml over 24 hours (2ml every hour is 24 lots of 2ml). What if I fill a syringe with 20ml fluid and set the rate of the pump to 4ml/hr? How many hours would it take for the fluid to be administered?

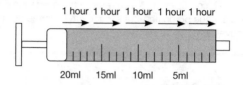

Figure 23 A syringe showing 20mls set at 4ml/hr

Every hour 4ml is infused, so two hours it would be 8ml, three hours 12ml, four hours 16ml and five hours 20ml. So the fluid would all be administered after five hours.

> **Warning!**
> The syringe pump doesn't know how much fluid is in the syringe, it only knows to keep administering the number of millilitres you ask it to every hour. We have to ensure that there is sufficient volume in the syringe so that it continues for the prescribed 24 hours. If you set it at the wrong rate, then the syringe may still contain fluid at the end or be empty before the 24 hours is up. Don't blame the syringe pump; it's only doing what you asked it to do!

So far we have learnt that a syringe pump administers a set amount of millilitres of fluid per hour according to the amount it is programmed. In order for fluid to be administered over the 24-hour prescription time, there needs to be sufficient volume of fluid in the syringe and the rate set correctly. We have demonstrated that a volume of 24ml set at 1ml/hr and 48ml set at 2ml/hr would allow a continuous infusion over 24 hours. Similarly, you could have 12ml of fluid set at 0.5ml/hr or 36ml set at 1.5ml/hr (0.5ml multiplied by 24 = 12ml and 1.5 multiplied by 24 = 36ml).

If you are feeling this is a little complex, then I have some good news for you. In clinical practice, there is generally a convention for syringe pumps. This is that a 50ml syringe is used and the volume administered is 48ml (n.b. 2ml used for priming infusion line). In practice, this means that in order to have a continuous infusion using a syringe pump over 24 hours, the rate of the pump needs to be set at 2ml/hr. Phew!

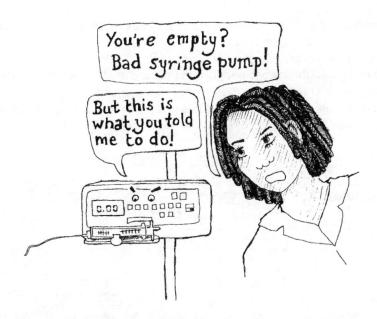

It is useful to be confident and know the frequent multiples of 12 and 24 for syringe pumps and syringe drivers since they are set per hour over 24 hours but sometimes 12 hourly. The useful multiples to know are:

2 × 12 = 24	2 × 24 = 48
3 × 12 = 36	3 × 24 = 72
4 × 12 = 48	4 × 24 = 96

What we haven't mentioned yet is the actual medication! Now the prescriptions are usually written as a set dosage to be infused over 24 hours. Previously, we used the example of 25 000 units of heparin so I'll continue with this.

Heparin ampoules contain different strengths of heparin in 1ml fluid. Instead of weight per volume, the dose for heparin is expressed as units per volume. This does not make any difference to how you calculate except that the number is a lot bigger to deal with!

A 25 000 unit heparin ampoule contains 25 000 units dissolved in 1ml. If we were to use this on its own for a syringe pump, we would have great difficulty in trying to infuse 1ml continuously over 24 hours. This would be approximately 0.042ml per hour! In addition to the practicalities, drugs administered directly into a patient's vein can cause irritation and inflammation so dilution is preferred.

Using the convention of a 50ml syringe the 25 000 units/1ml would be drawn up into the syringe and then the volume made up to 50ml in total with sodium chloride 0.9%. This syringe now contains 25 000 units/50ml. Although you don't need to know this just now, you will as we move on! (See Figure 24.)

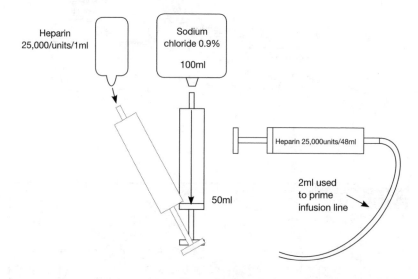

Figure 24 Illustration of how to set up the syringe for a syringe pump

Remember, in the tips for learning, I explained that 2ml of fluid is necessary to prime the infusion line? So if we prime the infusion line using the 50ml volume, this leaves 48ml in the syringe. When this is attached to the pump the rate can be set to ensure a continuous amount of heparin is administered every hour.

Warning!
Although the convention is to use a 50ml syringe and set the rate as 2ml/hr for a 48ml infusion, you should always check the syringe pump to ensure that it is set to the right rate and ensure that you always understand what it is you are calculating and how the infusion works over the 24 hours.

Let's work through another example together before I give you some infusions to work out yourself. The prescription is for 40 000 units of heparin over 24 hours and the heparin ampoules are 50 000 units/1ml.

Firstly, you will need to calculate what volume of the ampoule contains 40 000 units and then add this to the 50ml syringe. This is the same as the weight/volume calculations we did in the previous chapter for injections, but with bigger numbers! You can do this in different ways:

(a) Look at the pattern between 40 000 and 50 000. You may see that this is four-fifths and you therefore need four-fifths of 1ml, which is 0.8ml

(b) You may draw up the 50 000 units into a 1ml syringe and see that every 0.1ml graduation is 5000 units so you need to administer 0.8ml

(c) You may use the formula to calculate 40 000 divided by 50 000 multiplied by 1ml = 0.8ml

You need 0.8ml of the 50 000 units/1ml heparin ampoule. This is added to a 50ml syringe and then the syringe is made up to 50ml volume using sodium chloride 0.9% (see Figure 24). The rate for the syringe pump would be 2ml/hr.

Procedure to follow:

1. Ensure you understand what it is the question is asking you to calculate.

2. Calculate the amount of the ampoule(s) that contains the prescribed dosage.

3. Check that this amount makes sense logically using your practice experience.

4. Place this volume of the ampoule(s) into a 50ml syringe with a leur lock (n.b. a 'leur lock' is a syringe with a screw-like mechanism on the end which twists and locks onto infusion lines, see Figure 7, Chapter 2).

5. Draw up 0.9% sodium chloride into the syringe to give a total of 50ml.

6. Complete a label detailing contents of syringe and attach this to syringe.

7. Attach the infusion line and prime this. You now have 48ml in your syringe.

8. Place syringe into the syringe pump and set rate for 2ml/hour.

EXERCISE 27

1. You need to set up an infusion of heparin 15 000 units over 24 hours. Calculate the amount of heparin required from the stock ampoules available of 25 000 units/1ml and the rate per hour for the syringe pump.
2. You need to set up an infusion containing 80mg dopamine hydrochloride in 50ml. The ampoules available are 40mg/ml. How many ampoules would you need?
3. A patient requires a heparin infusion drawn up of 20 000 units in 50ml over 24 hours. The ampoules available are 25 000 units/ml. How many millilitres of the available ampoule will you need to draw up? The infusion is set for 2ml/hr.

(Answers: page 228)

● **Dosage per Hour**

In some clinical settings where patients are clinically unstable, the dose of drugs may be required to be administered more precisely, for example high dependency units, intensive care units or neonatal units. In these situations, the exact amount of drug needs to be known every hour so that more precise monitoring and adjustment can be done according to the patient's condition.

Before, I mentioned that the total amount of volume and drug dosage in the syringe would be relevant and this is the reason why. Let's use an example from before and take this in steps to calculate the dose per hour.

Step 1
We have made up a 50ml syringe containing 40 000 units of heparin. The strength of solution is 40 000 units/50ml. Firstly, we need to work out how many units are contained in 1ml of this solution. This is similar to the reducing down to a single unit method we went through in Chapter 2:

50ml	40 000 units	
5ml	4000 units	divide by 10
1ml	800 units	divide by 5

Alternatively, you can divide the dose by the volume to find how many units are in 1ml. This would be 40 000 units ÷ 50ml = 800 units/1ml.

Step 2
Secondly, we need to know what rate the patient is receiving the infusion at, that is, ml per hour, and then use this to multiply the units/ml. So if this

infusion was set up at 2ml/hr, the patient would be receiving 2 lots of 800 units which would be 1600 units of heparin every hour.

To make this easier there is a formula that is used. Before throwing yourself with relief on this formula to save your brain from exploding, please ensure that you understand what it is the formula is helping you to calculate, that is, the dosage per hour of an infusion:

$$\frac{\text{total dosage to be infused}}{\text{volume of infusion}} \times \text{rate of infusion (ml/hr)} = \text{dosage per hour}$$

If we use this formula to calculate the above problem, we would set up the calculation as:

$$\frac{40\ 000\ \text{units}}{50\text{ml}} \times 2\text{ml/hr} = 1600\ \text{units every hour}$$

So you can see there are two ways you can work out the dosage per hour for a patient:

1. You can think through logically what it is that you are trying to work out and calculate the dosage per hour in two stages:
   (a) Work out the dosage per 1ml
   (b) Multiply the dosage for 1ml by number of millilitres patient is receiving every hour
2. You can use the formula.

As you would expect, though, I would recommend that initially you practise using the first method until you are sure that you understand what it is you are actually trying to calculate. It would also be beneficial for you to try to do these questions without using a calculator, as again it will help you to 'see' what it is you are actually doing.

Once you are clear clinically about the calculation, then you can move to using the formula. Use the first method to calculate the following exercise and then use your calculator and the formula to check your answer to the second part of each question (b).

✔ **Tips for Learning**

To help you keep the clinical context of the calculation in your mind as you solve the calculation, try writing what the numbers actually represent in the calculation that you've set up from the formula, that is, instead of writing 50, write 50ml. I would also suggest that you write the formula down in full first, including the context of what the number of the solution means, that is, dosage per hour. This helps you to keep your calculation close to the clinical context of what it is you are trying to work out and stops you becoming lost in the world of arbitrary numbers.

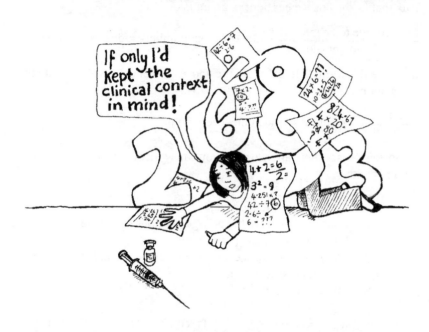

EXERCISE 28

1. Your patient requires 25mg of a drug in 50ml infused at a rate of 2ml/hr.
   - (a) How many milligrams does 1ml of the infusion contain?
   - (b) How many milligrams will the patient receive every hour?
2. You need to administer 50 000 units of heparin in 50ml to your patient at a rate of 4ml/hr.
   - (a) How many units does 1ml of the infusion contain?
   - (b) How many units of the drug will your patient receive every hour?
3. You set up an insulin infusion containing 50 units/50ml at a rate of 2ml/hr.
   - (a) How many units does 1ml of the infusion contain?
   - (b) How many units are being administered every hour?
4. You are required to set up an infusion containing 30 000 units of heparin in 50ml at a rate of 2ml/hr.
   - (a) How many units does 1ml of the infusion contain?
   - (b) How many units per hour is the patient receiving?

5.   You set up an infusion of dopamine containing 80mg/50ml and set the
      rate as 2ml/hr.
      (a)   How many milligrams does 1ml of the infusion contain?
      (b)   How many milligrams of the drug is the patient receiving per hour?

(Answers: page 229)

Sliding Scales

When a patient is clinically unstable, some drug dosages need to be administered according to the patient's clinical condition and altered to match this. This is especially important in clinical areas such as intensive care or neonatal units where drug dosages are finely adjusted according to the patient's clinical observations and condition. In these cases, drugs are often prescribed as a dosage range which is linked to a patient's specific clinical observation. This means that the dosage of the drug can be altered within the range depending on the individual patient.

For example, when a patient with diabetes requires their blood glucose levels to be finely controlled, for instance if these are unstable as a result of surgery, then they will be prescribed an insulin infusion with a dose of insulin given as a sliding scale. This means that the rate of the infusion is set according to the patient's blood glucose level. In practice, the patient's blood glucose is monitored every hour and the infusion rate varied according to the sliding scale prescribed. An example of a sliding scale for insulin can be seen in Box 17.

Box 17   An example of an insulin sliding scale

Blood glucose (mmol/L)	Insulin infusion rate (ml/hr)
0.4	0.5
4.1–7	1
7.1–11	2
11.1–15	3
15.1–20	4
< 20	6 and call doctors to review scale

The standard infusion set up for insulin is always 50 units Insulin Actrapid in 50ml 0.9% sodium chloride. Using this infusion, can you work out how many units of insulin the patient would be receiving for each of the rates above? (It won't take you long once you start working this out – try it and see!)

With the infusion of 50ml/50 units insulin, we can work out that 1ml will always contain 1 unit of insulin. Therefore the ml/hr rate above is easily worked out by multiplying this rate by 1 for the number of insulin units. You will basically be administering 0.5, 1, 2, 3, 4, 5 or 6 units of insulin per hour with this sliding scale prescription.

Quick question:
Your patient requires an infusion of insulin 50 units actrapid/50ml. If your patient's blood glucose level is 12mmol/L, what rate would you set this infusion up for using the sliding scale in Box 17 (ml/hr).

Answer:
50 units/50ml means that 1 unit/1ml. The patient requires 3 units of insulin with a blood glucose reading of 12mmol/L so the infusion should be set for 3ml/hr.

There are other scales that are used for certain drugs, but these are prescribed according to the patient's weight and are therefore more complicated. We shall be looking at these next.

● Infusion Dosages per Weight

In Chapter 2, we discussed the calculations required for drugs that are prescribed according to the patient's weight. This is the same with infusions. When the dosage calculated is given as a bolus dose, the drug is prescribed as a dosage per patient weight. With continuous infusions, however, the dosage needs to be moderated more finely to ensure the continuous administration of a set amount of drug in a set volume of fluid every minute.

This means that there are a number of stages to this calculation and naturally this makes the calculation slightly more complicated! Do not despair though. Once we break the calculation down and you understand what it is you are trying to calculate, it will be as simple to you as A B C. Deep breath …

The prescription for a drug will state, for example, 0.1mg/kg/min. This means:

- The dosage of the drug per kilogram weight of the patient
- This dosage needs to be administered to the patient every minute

(Let's look on the bright side; it could be worse, it could be per second of the infusion!)

Generally in specialist units such as ICU, the dosage will be given in a range such as 0.02–1.5mcg/kg/min. Thankfully most drugs and the dosages are given regularly and clinical areas have developed standard dosages and volumes for particular drugs to make calculations and administration of these drugs easier.

Let's go back to what we are trying to do clinically for a moment. We need to ensure that a patient receives a specific dosage of a drug every minute according to their weight. As syringe pumps deliver a set volume (ml) every hour, then we need to work out what volume administered every hour would contain the dosage required. (This dosage delivered continuously over the 60 minutes in the hour would give the amount required per minute.) The answer we are trying to calculate then is the ml/hr to set the syringe pump rate.

✱ Clinical Context

There are different methods of infusing these drugs to ensure the correct dosage is given depending on the area you work in. Some clinical areas use volumetric pumps and others use syringe pumps. You need to ensure that you are familiar with the method which is used in your own particular area. Despite these differences, the same principle for the calculation applies.

Step 1

First of all we can work out how much of the drug we require every minute according to the patient's weight. If the patient weighted 50kg and we are starting with the smallest dosage of 0.02mcg, then the dosage per minute would be 50kg × 0.02mcg = 1mcg. In order to work out the dosage per hour, we need to multiply this number by 60 (60 minutes in 1 hour) to get 60mcg per hour.

Step 2

Okay, now we need to pause and set up a syringe that contains the drug and a set volume. Once we have done this, we can use this to continue with the calculation. The standard amount for this drug in our clinical area is 4mg/50ml placed in a syringe pump.

Step 3

From this we can work out the dosage per millilitre. First, we need to convert milligrams to micrograms, otherwise the number will become too small: 4mg is the same as 4000mcg (multiplying by 1000). We now have 4000mcg/50ml. To work out how many micrograms in 1ml, you would divide 4000mcg by 50ml to get 80 micrograms:

4000mcg in 50ml
80mcg in 1ml (dividing both sides by 50)
Or 4000mcg ÷ 50ml = 80mcg/1ml

✔ **Tips for Learning**

Remember a previous tip of pretending that 4000 is really 40 and 50 is really 5, so you are calculating 40 divided by 5. This makes it easier to work out that it is 8 and then put the zeros back on that you took off before.

Step 4

Now we know that every 1ml contains 80mcg. If we set the syringe pump to administer 1ml/hr, the patient would receive 80mcg/hr. However, we need to give 60mcg every hour so we need to work out how many millilitres would give 60mcg by dividing this by 80mcg:

$$\frac{60}{80} = \frac{3}{4} = 0.75\text{ml/hr}$$

✔ **Tips for Learning**

What you're actually doing is working out what part of 60mcg is 80mcg. This can be done by writing it as a fraction, which is $^{60}/_{80}$, or by mentally dividing 80mcg into four equal 20mcg parts and recognising that 60mcg is three out of a potential four of these parts. 60mcg is therefore three-quarters, which is the same as 0.75ml.

Now, obviously, if you had to do this every time you needed to administer a drug in this way, you wouldn't have time for much else! So there are quicker ways that have been developed in clinical practice for calculating and administering these types of drugs.

Summarising this into stages, we have:

1. Ensure you understand what it is the question is asking you to calculate.
2. Calculate dose per weight of the patient: dosage/kg × patient's weight (kg).
3. Multiply the dose for the patient per minute by 60 to work out dosage per hour for this patient.
4. Convert usual infusion dose to micrograms.
5. Calculate dosage per millilitre using the usual infusion amounts: dose in infusion ÷ volume of infusion.
6. Calculate ml/hr: dosage per hour (answer to step 3 above) ÷ dosage in 1ml (answer to step 5 above).
7. Check your answer by repeating calculation, using clinical experience or logic to ensure 100% certainty before administering drug.

Example

Your patient has been prescribed 0.04mcg/kg/min of adrenaline. The infusion used in your area is 4mg/50ml. The patient's weight is 60kg. Calculate the rate per hour you would need to set this infusion up.

1. *Ensure you understand what it is the question is asking you to calculate:*

   Need to calculate how many mls/hr will contain the specific dose for my patient

2. *Calculate dose per weight of the patient: dosage/kg × patient's weight (kg):*

   0.04mcg × 60kg = 2.4mcg

3. *Multiply the dose for the patient per minute by 60 to work out dosage per hour for this patient:*

   2.4mcg × 60 = 144mcg

4. *Convert usual infusion dose to micrograms:*

   4mg × 1000 = 4000mcg/50ml

5. *Calculate dosage per millilitre using the infusion amounts: dose in infusion ÷ volume of infusion:*

$4000mcg \div 50ml = 80mg$

6. *Calculate ml/hr: dosage per hour ÷ dosage in 1ml:*

   $144mg \div 80mg = 1.8ml/hr$

7. *Check your answer by repeating calculation, using clinical experience or logic to ensure 100% certainty before administering drug.*

✔ Tips for Learning

These calculations are far quicker to do using a calculator and, for once, I would not recommend that you try to calculate the whole of this calculation using arithmetic (unless you particularly want to!). These types of calculations are commonly required in intensive care settings and high dependency units where you may have over 10 different infusions being administered to a patient at once. In these situations, there simply isn't time to work all these calculations out manually and you need to develop the skills of using your calculator and checking the solutions obtained.

Formula

These steps can be summarised into formulas:

- **Formula one** – depends on you knowing how to calculate dose per hour and dose per 1ml. If you are unsure then use formula two.

  $$\frac{\text{Dose per hour}}{\text{Dose in 1ml}} = ml/hr$$

- **Formula two**

  $$[\text{dose/kg} \times \text{patient weight (kg)} \times 60] \div \left[\frac{\text{dose in infusion}}{\text{volume of infusion}}\right] = ml/hr$$

? Maths Explained

The brackets mean that you complete the calculation contained within each bracket separately.

✔ Tips for Learning

Because most intensive care and high dependency units standardise their infusion amounts for specific drugs, the second part of the formula often remains constant. For example, if the infusion was always 4mg/50ml, for a specific drug, the amount per 1ml would be known immediately as 80mcg/1ml. This means that you need only calculate the first part of the formula and then divide this by the known amount per ml.

✔ Tips for Learning

When you are using the formula, it is always a good idea to write down on a piece of paper what the solution to each part of the calculation is. In addition to this I also recommend that you don't just write the number but also say what this number represents. For example, you could write:

dose per weight per hour = 420mcg
dose per 1ml = 240mcg
rate (ml/hr) = 420mcg ÷ 240mcg = 1.75 = 1.8ml/hr (rounded up to one decimal place)

The principle of these calculations remains the same whatever infusion volume is used to administer the drug. For some drugs, clinical areas may choose to have larger infusion volumes which are administered using volumetric pumps. These infusions are still set at millilitres per hour rate.

EXERCISE 29

1. Your patient has been prescribed 0.08mcg/kg/min of a drug. The patient weighs 65kg and the infusion used in your unit is 4mg/50ml. What rate per hour would you set this infusion up for?
2. Your patient needs to be administered 0.1mcg/kg/min of a drug. Your patient's weight is 70kg. The infusion used in your area is 12mg/50ml. Calculate the rate per hour you would set this infusion up for.
3. You need to administer 1mcg/kg/min of a drug. The infusion available is 800mg/500ml and your patient weights 48kg. How many millilitres per hour would you set this infusion for?

4. The prescription for your patient is 5mcg/kg/min of a drug. Your patient weighs 78kg and the standard infusion for your area is 200mg/50ml. What rate would you set this infusion for?
5. You need to administer 3mcg/kg/min of a drug. The infusion available is 250mg/50ml and your patient weighs 90kg. What rate would you set this infusion at?

(Answers:page 229)

Warning!
One of the complications of calculating these infusion rates is the conversion between different units of measurements that you need to do between the prescription dose and the dose in the infusion solution. You need to be aware of this complication and ensure that you are checking each time what unit of measurement your solution to any calculation is in.

There is another way that these calculations can be worked out. This method is similar to the formula we have used so far, but uses a principle that we covered in Chapter 2 in how to solve volume and weight calculations. The formula is:

$$\frac{\text{what you want to administer}}{\text{what you have available}} \times \text{volume it is dissolved in}$$

Where what you want to administer needs to be calculated by using:

dose per kg × patient weight (kg) × 60

So the formula is:

$$\frac{\text{dose per kg} \times \text{patient weight (kg)} \times 60}{\text{what you have available (dose in syringe, mcg)}} \times \text{volume it's dissolved in}$$

= rate per hour (ml/hr)

Some nurses find this formula easier to use and remember. When using a calculator, this formula is easier as you do not need to do any separate calculations just put the numbers and the operations straight into the calculator. For example, if you needed to administer 5mcg/kg/min of a drug with a standard infusion of 200mg/50ml and the patient weighed 56kg, the calculation you would set up would be:

$$\frac{5\text{mcg} \times 56\text{kg}}{200\ 000\text{mcg}^*} \times 60 \times 50 = 4.2\text{ml/hr}$$

* Because the prescription dose is in micrograms, I need to convert 200mg into micrograms so I have the same units of measurement in my calculation.

As a method for solving these calculations, I have put this formula last for two reasons. The first is that by the time you get to this point in the explanations I have given, the context of what you are trying to do clinically should be clearer. And, secondly, as a consequence of this, the formula above makes more sense and is more memorable. I did have reasons, honest, I wasn't just stringing you along!

● Syringe Drivers

Syringe drivers are very different from syringe pumps, although they have similarities in that they both continuously infuse over either 12 or 24 hours. The syringe pump works by slowly depressing a syringe a set **volume** of fluid per hour. The syringe driver works in the same way with a syringe being slowly depressed by the driver, but the rate is set according to the **length** of the syringe that is depressed. Syringe drivers are usually for medication administered subcutaneously, whereas syringe pumps are usually for intravenous medication (see Box 18).

Box 18 Similarities and differences between a syringe pump and a syringe driver

	Syringe pump	Syringe driver
Infusion time	Usually 12 or 24 hours	Usually 12 or 24 hours
Rate infused	Volume (ml) per hour	Length (mm) per hour or 24 hours
Infusion route	Intravenous	Subcutaneous (most often)

The main manufacturers of the syringe driver currently in use are Graseby. Graseby have two types of syringe drivers, which we will look at now:

● The first is programmed to infuse a certain length **per hour**
● The second is programmed to infuse a certain length **per 24 hours**

Warning!
Obviously it is important that you know which syringe driver you are using to ensure that you set the rate correctly. As a result of the confusion between the two syringe drivers, most clinical areas will use only one type of syringe driver so errors can be reduced.

✳ Clinical Context

Graseby was the most popular syringe driver in clinical areas up until recently. Some clinical areas are now beginning to use other manufacturers of syringe drivers rather than Graseby. For example, the T34 Ambulatory Syringe Pump manufactured by McKinley is starting to be used. More details can be found on their website.

Hourly syringe drivers (also known as Graseby MS16)

The driver can be programmed to infuse a certain length of the syringe every **hour**. Most often, syringe drivers are set up to infuse over 24 hours. The syringe driver measures the rate in millimetres per hour (mm/hr). Therefore, if you programmed the syringe driver to infuse a rate of 1mm/hr, you would need 24mm length of volume in your syringe. If you set the rate for 2mm/hr, the length of volume of the syringe would be 48mm. With an hourly syringe driver, the standard practice is to use a 10ml syringe and make the volume length up to 48mm (see Figure 25)

✔ Tips for Learning

The volume being infused isn't particularly important and it is not necessary to know how much of a particular drug a patient is receiving every hour with a syringe driver. What is important is that a continuous amount of the infusion, and the drugs it contains, is administered over the 12-hour or 24-hour period. We are therefore only interested in the 24-hour dose and ensuring that this is administered continually over the 24-hour period.

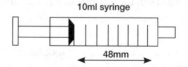

Figure 25 Diagram showing a 10ml syringe with the volume measuring 48mm for a syringe driver

Patients are often prescribed a number of drugs that need to be infused via a syringe driver over 24 hours. Like a syringe pump, these drugs need to be drawn up into the 10ml syringe and the volume made up with water for injection so that it measures 48mm. Thankfully there is a ruler on the front of the syringe driver to help! An example may make this clearer.

Your patient has been prescribed the following drugs to be given subcutaneously over 24 hours:

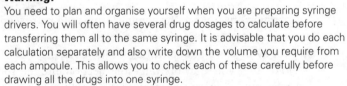

30mg morphine
5mg metoclopramide
600mcg hyoscine hydrobromide
} administered over 24 hours
via a syringe driver

To administer these drugs you need to follow several stages:

1. You need to calculate how much of the available ampoule for each drug you would administer (this is the same procedure for calculating weight/volume dosages covered in Chapter 2).
2. The appropriate volume of each drug ampoule needs to be drawn up into a 10ml syringe.
3. The volume in the syringe is then made up until it equals the **length** 48mm.

> **Warning!**
> You need to plan and organise yourself when you are preparing syringe drivers. You will often have several drug dosages to calculate before transferring them all to the same syringe. It is advisable that you do each calculation separately and also write down the volume you require from each ampoule. This allows you to check each of these carefully before drawing all the drugs into one syringe.

We will go through each of the stages with the example given:

Worked through example

1. Calculating the dosage for each drug prescribed:
   (a) 30mg morphine sulphate has been prescribed. Stock ampoules available are 30mg/2ml. We therefore need to draw up the whole 2ml ampoule
   (b) 5mg metoclopramide has been prescribed. The stock ampoules available are 10mg/2ml. Therefore you need to draw up half of the ampoule, which would be 1ml. If you haven't followed this, then try the halving method:

10mg in 2ml
5mg in 1ml (halving)

(c) 600mcg hyoscine has been prescribed. The ampoules available are 400mcg/1ml. You can calculate the amount to administer by using halving techniques:

400mcg in 1ml
200mcg in 0.5ml

So you need to administer one lot of 400mcg (1ml) and one lot of 200mcg (0.5ml): in total this is 1.5ml. Or you can use the formula method:

$$\frac{600mg}{400mg} \times 1ml = 1.5ml$$

Therefore you need to administer 1.5ml.

2. Now you have the drugs you want to administer drawn up in three different syringes:
    - 2ml morphine sulphate containing 30mg
    - 1ml metoclopramide containing 5mg
    - 1.5ml hyoscine containing 600mg
    You can now add these three drug dosages to a 10ml syringe.

3. The syringe driver works by administering millimetre lengths of the syringe per hour so you need to ensure that the total length in your syringe is a multiple of 24 for the 24 hours.

    To do this, you draw up water for injection into the 10ml syringe containing your drugs until the length of volume you have is a multiple of 24. You can either use a ruler or the measurements on the front of the syringe driver.

    For simplicity and to avoid confusion and error, most hourly syringe drivers are set at a rate of 2mm/hr and the syringe filled to a length of 48mm.

✳ Clinical Context

In practice, you probably wouldn't see nurses drawing up each drug separately into three syringes and then decanting these into the 10ml syringe. As you become more experienced at setting up syringe drivers and learn the compatibilities of different drugs, you can use some short cuts to the drawing up the drug dose process.

For the above example, you know you need 1ml of metoclopramide so you can draw this up first into a 10ml syringe. You can then draw up the hyoscine, so you now have a total volume of 3ml. You can then draw up the whole ampoule to make 5ml.

The steps we have gone through here are:

1. Ensure that you understand what it is you are calculating.
2. For each drug, calculate the required volume that contains the prescribed dose.
3. Confirm that each calculation is correct through recalculating to check, and using your clinical experience and logic.
4. Draw up each drug either separately and add to a 10ml leur lock syringe or straight into a 10ml leur lock syringe.
5. Make up the volume in the 10ml syringe by drawing up water for injection to a length of 48mm.
6. Ensure that the syringe driver is an hourly syringe driver and that the rate is set for 2mm/hr.

Follow these steps in the example below:

Example

Prescription		Stock ampoules available
30mg morphine sulphate	administered over	60mg/2ml morphine sulphate
10mg midazolam	24 hours via a	10mg/1ml midazolam
2.5mg haloperidol	syringe driver	5mg/1ml haloperidol

1. *Ensure that you understand what it is you are calculating:*

   Need to add each of the required drugs into a 10ml syringe and make up the volume to a length of 48mm to put into a syringe driver

2. *For each drug, calculate the required volume that contains the prescribed dose:*

   - morphine sulphate

   Use halving, patterns between prescribed and available dose or formula to solve calculation:

(a)   60mg in 2ml

        30mg in 1ml (halving)

(b)   30mg is half of 60mg so you need half of 2ml, which is 1ml

(c) $\dfrac{30mg}{60mg} \times 2ml = 1ml$

- midazalam

Use the whole ampoule to administer 10mg

- haloperidol

Use halving method to calculate that you need half of the ampoule to administer 2.5mg, which is 0.5ml

3.   *Confirm that each calculation is correct through recalculating to check, and using your clinical experience and logic:*

morphine sulphate 60mg/2ml, so logically 30mg would be half the whole ampoule which is 1ml

midazolom 10mg/1ml, so draw up the whole ampoule

haloperidol 5mg/1ml, so 2.5 mg in 0.5ml is logical

4.   *Draw up each drug either separately and add to a 10ml syringe or straight into a 10ml syringe:*

If unsure draw each drug up separately and then add to a 10ml syringe

5.   *Make up the volume in the 10ml syringe to a length of 48mm using water for injection:*

Use the ruler on syringe driver or own ruler to carefully draw up the volume so that it measures a length of 48mm

6.   *Ensure that the syringe driver is an hourly syringe driver and that rate is set for 2mm/hr.*

Warning!
Some drugs are not compatible to be mixed together in a syringe driver. Most clinical areas will have a list of drugs that are compatible available for reference. Compatibilities must be checked before drawing up the drugs into a syringe.

Warning!
If the solution becomes cloudy or crystallises when you have drawn up the drugs, then the solution needs to be discarded and the compatibility of the drugs rechecked. If in doubt seek advice.

Variations

There are times when the dosage, and hence the volume of drugs, that the patient requires is very large and is greater than the 48mm length of a 10ml syringe. When this happens there are several things that we can do:

1. We could draw the drugs up into a 20ml syringe. The 48mm length of a 20ml syringe contains more volume than a 10ml syringe since it is wider. You do not need to change anything in the process of setting this up except for the size of the syringe.
2. We could calculate the drug dosage for 12 hours and set the syringe to run over 12 hours instead of 24 hours. In this case we would halve all the drugs and draw them up into either a 10ml or a 20ml syringe depending on volume.

    We would make the volume up to the 48mm as before but, as we want the driver to administer the drugs over half the time, we need to change the rate that the syringe driver is set at. If we want all of the 48mm volume length to be administered in 12 hours, what rate do we need to change the driver to? To work this out we divide the length by the hours, so it is 48mm divided by 12 hours, which is a rate of 4mm/hr.

Warning!
Only in exceptional circumstances should the syringe driver rate be altered. Where possible it is better to try to remain with the standard 2mm/hr rate and change the size of the syringe.

✱ Clinical Context

If you are ever in any doubt about setting up a syringe driver, there is always a member of your local palliative care team on call (either at a local hospice or hospital) who you can ring and check your calculation and administration rates with.

EXERCISE 30

Using the prescriptions below, calculate the volume of each medicine required in the syringe and describe how you would draw these up to administer using a 24-hour syringe driver.

1. Prescription		Stock ampoules available
morphine sulphate 120mg midazolam 10mg levomepromazine 50mg	administered over 24 hours via a syringe driver	morphine sulphate 60mg/ml midazolam 10mg/2ml levomepromazine 25mg/1ml

2. Prescription		Stock ampoules available
morphine sulphate 20mg cyclizine 75mg haloperidol 10mg	administered over 24 hours via a syringe driver	morphine 20mg/1ml cyclizine 50mg/1ml haloperidol 5mg/1ml

3. Prescription		Stock ampoules available
morphine sulphate 240mg midazolam 20mg hyoscine hydrobromide 0.6mg	administered over 24 hours via a syringe driver	morphine sulphate 60mg/ml midazolam 10mg/2ml hyoscine hydrobromide 400mcg/1ml

4. Prescription		Stock ampoules available
morphine sulphate 30mg haloperidol 2.5mg	administered over 24 hours via a syringe driver	morphine sulphate 30mg/ml haloperidol 5mg/1ml

5. Prescription		Stock ampoules available
morphine sulphate 180mg hyoscine butylbromide 60mg	administered over 24 hours via a syringe driver	morphine sulphate 60mg/2ml hyoscine butylbromide 20mg/1ml

(Answers: page 229)

24-hour syringe drivers (Graseby MS26)

So far we have talked about the 1-hour syringe drivers. There is another syringe driver available that is identical to the Graseby 1-hour driver, but it is green rather than blue and most importantly it administers the volume in the syringe according to the rate for the **whole 24 hours**.

The hourly syringe driver administered the volume according to the rate per hour so that if you programmed it to administer '2', it would administer 2mm of volume every hour. The 24-hour syringe driver, though, administers the length you set the rate at over the total 24-hour period. So if you programmed in '2', it would only administer 2mm over the 24 hours!

For the 24-hour syringe driver, therefore, the rate is set according to the length of volume you want to give over the **whole 24-hour period**. If you had a volume measuring 48mm, then you would set up the rate as 48.

Warning!
You can probably start to see what the major problems could be if you work in an area that uses both types of syringe driver. If you set a syringe driver up with an administration rate of 48mm/hr, thinking it was a 24-hour driver, but it was actually an hourly driver, the patient would be administered the whole syringe in 1 hour! It makes perfect sense then that most areas will only use one type of syringe driver.

Chapter Summary

This chapter has explained the main calculations involving continuous infusions. We have looked at fluid replacement infusions and calculated how to administer these using a manual giving set and using a volumetric infusion device. We then looked at continuous infusions involving medications and explained the different types: dosages to be administered hourly using a syringe pump, and more complex calculations involving prescriptions of dosages per weight of the person per minute, administered in more acute settings such as ICU and neonatal units.

Finally, this chapter has explained administration of medication prescribed over 24 hours using a syringe driver, often used for palliative care. This chapter has covered a lot and much of it has built on the skills you learnt in Chapters 1 and 2. If you are not feeling confident, you may want to go over bits of this chapter or the previous two chapters again. If you are feeling confident, though, then have a go at Assessment 3.

Assessment 3

Use the IV medicine chart below to complete questions 1–3.

Sunnydene and Reynold NHS Trust

Intravenous medicine administration chart

Name: Fred Kumar   **Hospital Number:** 0789655   **Consultant:** Rogers

Date of Birth: 1/9/1952   **Ward:** Oak

Date prescribed	Solution	Volume	Duration of infusion	Date to be given	Prescriber's signature
1/2/2011	0.9% sodium chloride	1000ml	8 hours	1/2/2011	R Dickenson
1/2/2011	Blood	1 unit (0.5L)	4 hours	2/2/2011	R Dickenson
1/2/2011	4% glucose, 0.18% sodium chloride (dextrose saline)	500ml	8 hours	2/2/2011	R Dickenson

1. Using the IV medicine chart, calculate the infusion rate using a volumetric pump for the 0.9% sodium chloride.

2. Using the IV medicine chart, calculate the drip rate for the blood transfusion (giving set drop factor of 15drops/ml).

3. Using the IV medicine chart, calculate the number of grams of glucose in the dextrose saline infusion prescribed.

4. Your patient has been written up for the following prescription:

Prescription		Stock ampoules available
morphine sulphate 60mg	administered over 24 hours via a syringe driver	morphine sulphate 60mg/ml
midazolam 5mg		midazolam 10mg/2ml
levomepromazine 25mg		levomepromazine 25mg/1ml

Calculate the number of millilitres of the available stock ampoules for each drug. Using a 1-hour syringe driver, what rate (mm/hr) would you set this driver for?

5. You patient has been prescribed heparin 40 000 units/50ml over 24 hours. The stock ampoules of heparin available are 50 000 units/ml. How many millilitres of this ampoule would you need for the infusion? If you set this infusion rate as 2ml/hr, how many units of heparin would your patient be receiving every hour?

6. Your patient has been prescribed 1000ml 5% dextrose infusion over 12 hours. Using a manual giving set with a drop factor of 20 drops/ml, calculate what rate you would set this infusion for.

7. Your patient needs to be administered 0.2mcg/kg/min of a drug. Your patient's weight is 65kg. The infusion used in your area is 12mg/50ml. Calculate the rate per hour you would set this infusion up for.

8. You set up an infusion of dopamine containing 80mg/50ml and set the rate as 3ml/hr. How many milligrams of the drug is the patient receiving per hour?

9. Your patient has been prescribed 50 units actrapid/50ml and requires 4 units per hour administered initially. What rate would you set this infusion for?

10. You need to administer 1mcg/kg/min of a drug. The infusion available is 800mg/500ml and your patient weights 52kg. How many millilitres per hour would you set this infusion for?

(Answers: page 230)

Part II

Practice and assessment

4 Maths Fitness Programme! Practice, practice, practice

❝*The 'oops-I've-forgotten-my-maths!' step – to get you back to full maths fitness***❞**

● Introduction

In this chapter, I'm going to take you through a brief, but fun, tour of the maths you require for drug calculations! This section is divided into five sessions. I would advise that you plan to do one session every couple of days until you have completed your fitness programme.

Okay, so I said initially that you don't need pure maths in order to do drug calculations. That's true. However, as calculations involve numbers, you do need a basic understanding of numbers and how to manipulate them. Generally, you will gain this understanding through everyday interactions such as shopping and managing your money. However, the use of numbers in healthcare can sometimes be quite specific to the clinical context and you will need to understand their meanings and be able to quickly manipulate these, for example in drug calculations. Therefore, alongside your nursing skills you will need an understanding of numeracy.

If you are worried that I am going to launch into a maths lesson here, then be reassured that I'm not. I don't believe that this will help your drug calculations. I do believe, however, that if you can understand numbers in a clinical context and can see the relevance and meaning to any manipulation of numbers in relation to the patient and the care you are implementing, then this will help your calculation skills. For this reason, I have attempted to always relate the numeracy in this chapter to clinical practice so you can 'see' its relevance and to help you to make sense of what you are doing in a clinical context.

In order to manipulate numbers, you will need to either have sound arithmetic skills or have access to a calculator. As many assessments of nurses and student nurses' drug calculation skills can involve completing tests without calculators, then you will need to ensure that your basic arithmetic skills are sound. The NMC also stipulates that we all need to have sound numeracy skills and be able to solve calculations, if necessary, without a calculator.

Generally, the main mathematical knowledge you will need to solve drug calculations are the four main arithmetic processes of subtraction, addition, multiplication and division. Along with these you will need to have an understanding of place value, fractions, ratios, percentages and decimals.

At the beginning of this section you'll see a short maths test or assessment. This will help you to identify areas that you may need to work on to improve your numeracy skills.

Once you have completed the test, have a go at the maths fitness programme (or perhaps just the section that you need extra work on).

If you find that you are not clear about some of the areas in the fitness programme and you are still struggling, then I would advise you to take some time out and find a basic maths textbook which you can work through to help you. Please note, though, that you do not need any maths book above secondary/high school level.

● Test Your Maths Skills

Assessment

Please complete the following test to the best of your abilities. It is designed to help identify areas that you need to work on. Please do not use a calculator. Your marks for each question will give you feedback on your strengths and areas requiring further work.

Question 1

    (a) $125 + 500 =$
    (b) $150 + 120 =$
    (c) $62.5 + 125 =$
    (d) $500 + 1000 + 200 =$
    (e) $17 + 33 + 65 + 36 =$

Mark =

Question 2

    (a) $5 \times 50 =$
    (b) $125 \times 4 =$
    (c) $200 \times 8 =$
    (d) $100 \times 10 =$
    (e) $8 \times 125 =$

Mark =

Question 3

(a) ½ x ½ =
(b) ¾ x ½ =
(c) ¼ x ¼ =
(d) 8 x ¼ =
(e) ½ x 125 =

Mark =

Question 4

Express the following in decimals:

(a) ½
(b) ¾
(c) ⅕ (one-fifth)
(d) ⅒ (one-tenth)
(e) ⅖ (two-fifths)

Mark =

Question 5

(a) 1000 ÷ 10 =
(b) 250 ÷ 4 =
(c) 500 ÷ 25 =
(d) 1720 ÷ 8 =
(e) 5001 ÷ 3 =

Mark =

Question 6

(a) 10% of 1000 =
(b) 5% of 1000 =
(c) 10% of 500 =
(d) 15% of 200 =
(e) 0.9% of 1000 =

Mark =

Question 7

(a) 50 x 1000 =
(b) 1.8 x 1000 =
(c) 0.125 x 1000 =
(d) 5000 ÷ 1000 =
(e) 300 ÷ 1000 =

Mark =

Question 8

(a) 2500 − 500 =
(b) 1100 − 200 =
(c) 1245 − 1220 =
(d) 945 − 846 =
(e) 1288 − 1298 =

Mark =

Question 9

(a) What is ¼ of 100ml?

(b) What fraction is 250ml of 500ml?

(c) You need to administer 1000ml fluid over 10 hours. How many milli-litres (ml) would you administer per hour?

(d) Your patient has the following 2-hourly urine output over 12 hours: 55ml, 50ml, 62ml, 76ml, 45ml, 68ml. What is the total urine output for the 12 hours?

(e) Your patient's diastolic blood pressure was 68mmHg. When you recheck their blood pressure their diastolic reading is 95mmHg. How much has the diastolic pressure increased by?

Mark =

Question 10

(a) John requires 50mg of morphine. The morphine ampoules contain 100mg in 2ml. How many millilitres would you give?

(b) Jane has been prescribed 1000ml 0.9% sodium chloride to be infused over 8 hours. How many millilitres per hour would her infusion run?

(c) Midazalam ampoules contain 20mg in 2ml. You require 5mg. How much would you draw up?

(d) John requires 1.8g benzylpenicillin. Benzylpenicillin ampoules each contain 600mg. How many ampoules would you administer?

(e) Stacey has been prescribed 0.25mg digoxin. The digoxin tablets are 62.5mcg. How many tablets would you give?

Mark =

Total =

(Answers: page 232)

Feedback

The table below outlines the main areas that the questions covered. Have a look at how you did on these questions and consider how confident you felt working them out as well as whether you got the right answers. For example, you may have got the right answers to all the problems in Question 1, but are you sure about how you arrived at these answers? Perhaps you don't feel confident about the answers you worked out. As well as your mark, use your evaluation of each question in the assessment to decide whether you feel you would benefit from more practice in this area. See below for suggestions of sections of the chapter to work through for each area of maths covered in the above assessment.

Areas covered in each question	Sections to work through for more practice
Q1 Addition	Work through all of the maths fitness sessions
Q2 Multiplication	Work through all of the maths fitness sessions
Q3 Multiplication of fractions	Work through maths session two
Q4 Expressing fractions as decimals/long division	Work through maths session two
Q5 Division/long division	Work through maths sessions two and three
Q6 Percentages	Work through all the maths sessions
Q7 Place value	Work through maths session one
Q8 Subtraction	Work through maths sessions one and two
Q9 General numeracy/ word problems	Try to visualise what the question is asking you – pull out the numbers. Pay particular attention to the exercises which are given as word problems
Q10 Drug calculations	Focus on gaining practice experience and working through the chapters in this book, particularly Chapters 1–3

● Session One – Maths Fitness

Having completed the maths test, as you are now here, you have probably identified that your maths is an area you would like to develop. This is not an impossible task (although you may think it is). The first very easy step is to believe in yourself. People are not born either being able to do maths or not. The midwife did not turn to your mother when you were born and say 'congratulations you have a baby girl, but commiserations as she won't be able to do maths'! We can all develop our maths, whatever our current ability … but we will have to work at it and develop our maths fitness.

The first step in our maths fitness programme is potentially the most important one:

1. Believe you can do it!

If you keep repeating 'I'm no good at maths' or 'I can't do maths', as I've have heard people say, then this will become self-fulfilling. You won't be able to do maths and you won't be very good. You need to develop your confidence and change your thinking. You can do maths. Okay, you may not be as good as some other people, but you can do the basics (let's face it, if you couldn't, you wouldn't be able to handle money when you go shopping or know what speed limit you are supposed to be under when you are driving … no using your maths as an excuse for your overdraft or speeding fine though!). And, you are also willing to work on improving (after all, you are here and reading this). I once heard an athlete talking about how she focuses before she attempts different heights in high jump and she said she repeated the following phrase over and over in her mind 'I can and I will, I can and I will'. So you **can** do maths and with some work you **will** do it.

Okay, second step, which, like any fitness programme, will require a little effort:

2. Warm-up

In this step, we need to start jogging on the spot and chanting our times tables. No I'm not joking. This may take you straight back in your memories to horrible maths teachers yelling at you for getting the answer wrong or not knowing an answer, but it will be really useful for you to start seeing the patterns in numbers and will speed up your mental calculations no end (and anyway who's around now to see you if you get it wrong?). Okay … ready? Go to your starting place and start the times tables below.

Times table warm-up

Below is a table for you to copy and jog around to warm up, filling in each square with the number you get when you multiply the two numbers in the grey boxes together. By way of illustration, the square I have filled in as an example is the result of 4 multiplied by 3, or 3 multiplied by 4. Once you have completed the table you can display it on your fridge door or on the wall next to your toilet so you'll have a regular reminder! Or you could photocopy lots of the blank tables and post them around your house to complete when you have a dull moment! So are you ready to fill this in? Put on some music and off you go …

You can use a calculator if you must, but that would be like using a car to jog around the block! Have a go, you'll be amazed at how good you'll feel and how many interesting sights you'll see along the way. You can check your table with a similar table we've completed for you (see Answers: page 232). Having just returned from a little jaunt around the table myself, I would well recommend varying your direction along the table, sideways, from left to right and bottom to top. It gives those maths muscles a great work out!

Another little exercise you can try in pairs, which again gets those maths muscles working, is a matching the number game. To start with, your partner gives a number between 0 and 10. You then need to give the number that, when added to this number, will make 10. For example, if I said 4, you'd say 6. If I said 2, you'd say 8. The idea is to see if you can keep a rhythm going between you so it is short and snappy.

	1	2	3	4	5	6	7	8	9	10	11	12
1												
2												
3												
4			12									
5												
6												
7												
8												
9												
10												
11												
12												

NB: a blank version of this square is available at www.palgrave.com/nursinghealth/ wright).

(Answers: page 232)

Once you can do this, you can build up to flexing the big muscles and do the same exercise but this time giving a number between 0 and 100 and finding the partner number which, when added, will give 100. For example, if I said 45, you'd say 55. If I said 17, you'd say 83.

This is a great exercise that can be done anywhere and could while away a long train journey or fill in a few minutes while you're waiting in a queue with a friend.

3. Let's get started

Okay, so you're all warmed up from your exertions and ready to start.

During your warm-up you filled in the table with numbers and paired numbers which added up to 10 and 100. These types of numbers are called whole numbers. Whole numbers, as you would probably guess, are complete numbers for example 1, 2, 3, 4, 5, 6. Most people are quite comfortable with whole numbers as these are the numbers we generally deal with every day. For example, it is easy to add up £5 and £3. The difficulty comes when numbers aren't whole and have decimals or fractions to express their 'unwholeness'.

You can express the numbers 1 to 10 in the table below:

0	1	2	3	4	5	6	7	8	9	10

But you can also divide up the 'parts' between 0 and 1. Below we have divided 1 into 10 parts:

0	0.1	0.2	0.3	0.4	0.5	0.6	0.7	0.8	0.9	1

We could also divide up the 'parts' between 0 and 0.1 into 10 parts:

0	0.01	0.02	0.03	0.04	0.05	0.06	0.07	0.08	0.09	0.1

And again between 0 and 0.01:

0	0.001	0.002	0.003	0.004	0.005	0.006	0.007	0.008	0.009	0.01

Can you see any pattern developing? The top table represents the whole numbers. We then divided 1 number into 10 parts to get tenths. We then divided that number by 10 again to get the numbers in the third table and by 10 again, finally, to get the numbers in the fourth table. We could carry on dividing by 10 for as long as we liked, but I hope by now you can spot a pattern building up every time we divide by 10. What does the 'dot' do?

I'm sure you all know that the 'dot' is called the decimal point. Can you now see why it is called that? The 'Deci' bit means 10 (those who like athletics will know that the decathlon has 10 events) so the decimal point is dividing the whole number into units of 10.

I hope that you have spotted that every time you divide by 10 the decimal point moves one number to the left. If you didn't spot that have a look at the tables again. What would 0.004 divided by 10 be? You should have moved the decimal point another place to the left to get 0.0004.

The same principle applies when you increase numbers by 10. Look at these tables:

1	2	3	4	5	6	7	8	9	10
10	20	30	40	50	60	70	80	90	100
100	200	300	400	500	600	700	800	900	1000
1000	2000	3000	4000	5000	6000	7000	8000	9000	10 000
10 000	20 000	30 000	40 000	50 000	60 000	70 000	80 000	90 000	100 000

Each row has been multiplied by 10. What has happened to that number? Hopefully you should all say in a weary 'that's really obvious' tone that the numbers get an extra zero stuck on every time you multiply by 10. Now if you add in the decimal place that is in each of these numbers, but that no one can ever be bothered to write when it's a whole number, you should be able to see that it's not really just a zero being added, but that the decimal point is up to its old trick and is moving one number to the … which way? It was left when dividing? So this time we are **increasing** the number, so it's to the right.

So 1 would be 1.0. Look at the table below with the decimal point in:

1.0	2.0	3.0	4.0	5.0	6.0	7.0	8.0	9.0	10.0
10.0	20.0	30.0	40.0	50.0	60.0	70.0	80.0	90.0	100.0
100.0	200.0	300.0	400.0	500.0	600.0	700.0	800.0	900.0	1000.0
1000.0	2000.0	3000.0	4000.0	5000.0	6000.0	7000.0	8000.0	9000.0	10 000.0
10 000.0	20 000.0	30 000.0	40 000.0	50 000.0	60 000.0	70 000.0	80 000.0	90 000.0	100 000.0

Okay. We are almost finished for this session today. We don't want to overdo it on the first session so you end up with sore muscles and don't want to come back next time. To start warming down, do the short exercise here looking at multiplying and dividing by 10.

EXERCISE 31

1. 1 x 10 =
2. 10 x 10 =
3. 100 x 10 =
4. 6 x 10 =
5. 125 x 10 =

6. 1 ÷ 10 =
7. 10 ÷ 10 =
8. 100 ÷10 =
9. 70 ÷ 10 =
10. 1000 ÷ 10 =

(Answers: page 233)

So far we have demonstrated that if we want to divide by 10, we move the decimal point to the left and to multiply by 10, we move the decimal point to the right. What do we do then if you want to divide by 100? Bearing in mind that 10 x 10 is 100, you should all see that we would move the decimal point two places to the left. If we multiply by a 1000, we are effectively multiplying the number by 10 by 10 by 10 so we move the decimal point 1…2…3… places to the right. I hope now that the table below will make sense:

ten thousands	thousands	hundreds	tens	units	tenths	hundredths	thousandths

Using the table above we can begin to understand different numbers and what they mean within the place value system. The decimal place marks the point where numbers change from whole numbers to part of a whole number and we start to describe numbers as a tenth, a hundredth and so on, as we showed at the beginning.

For example, if we had the number 125 this could be written:

ten thousands	thousands	hundreds	tens	units	tenths	hundredths	thousandths
0	0	1	2	5	0	0	0

This means that there are no ten thousands, no thousands, 1 hundred, 2 tens, 5 units and no tenths, hundredths, or thousandths. By convention we would, though, write the number as 125. Using this principle can you put the following numbers into the chart below?

EXERCISE 32

Numbers:
1. 175
2. 1.4
3. 37
4. 0.125
5. 1000.25

Question	ten thousands	thousands	hundreds	tens	units	tenths	hundredths	thousandths
1								
2								
3								
4								
5								

(Answers: page 233)

Therefore, if you have followed me so far and haven't left the room in disgust, you should be able to say what each of the numbers, in the number below is representing:

12 345.678

Have a think first. Which number is representing the hundreds, which one the thousandths? Once you've had a go, check your answer here:

Place value

12 345. 678

12 = ten thousands ⎫ 1 ten thousand
⎭ 2 thousands

3 = hundreds
4 = tens
5 = units
6 = tenths
7 = hundredths
8 = thousandths

Putting it all together:

10 000.
2000
300.
40.
5.
0.600
0.070
0.008
12 345.678

Now at this point I need to explain what is really happening with the numbers when you increase or decrease their size by 10 or 100. (If you don't understand this don't worry, but it is important that I at least explain mathematically what is really happening to satisfy the picky mathematicians who may be checking this book!) When I explained that you were moving the decimal point a certain number of places to the left or the right, I wasn't strictly being truthful. When you look at the number and calculate increases and decreases that are tenfold or hundredfold, this is what you see happening: the decimal point is hopping and skipping one way or the other. Using the place value system above, though, we can see what is really happening when we do this. For example, imagine that we want to multiply 1.6 by 100. Look at what is happening in the place value diagram below:

	ten thousands	thousands	hundreds	tens	units	tenths	hundredths	thousandths
Number					1	6		
Multiply by 100			1	6	0	0		

What has actually happened is the number has moved two places along the number line to make it 160. So in actual fact it is the number that is moving, not the decimal place.

I think we've almost finished now. All that's left is for you to complete the assessment for this session to see whether you have followed it all then go and have a shower to wash all that sweat away after all your exertions! (It should go without saying that the idea is that you do the assessment without a calculator.)

✔ Tips for Learning

If you are dividing a number such as 2.45 by 1000, to make it easier for you to see where the decimal point is going try writing your number like this:

0002.45

It is now much clearer for you when you are counting 3 places left and moving the decimal point (your answer should have been 0.00245). The same principle applies if you are multiplying. For example, 13.5 multiplied by 100 000 should be written initially with some extra zeros:

13.500 000 000

Now you can hop skip and jump that little decimal point to the right five times to get the answer 1350 000.
Hope that helps a little.

Assessment Session One

1. Which of the following numbers are whole numbers?
   2   ½   1.5   10   125

2. How many parts does a decimal point divide a whole number into?

3. If you are multiplying or dividing a number by 1000, how many places would the decimal place move?

4. With the number 87.5 what do each of the numbers represent?

5. 100 x 10 =

6. 1500 ÷ 100 =

7. 0.125 x 1000 =

8. $1800 \div 1000 =$

9. $500 \div 1000 =$

10. $0.0625 \times 1000 =$

(Answers: page 233)

● Session Two – Maths Stamina

Welcome to session two in your five-session work out. I hope that by now you have had the opportunity to practise your maths in the exercises given in the last session and have got the old brain muscles back into action again. So, that being the case, you should be ready for the next step. Last session we went over decimal points and how to multiply and divide by tens, hundreds and thousands. You should now be competent at these and be able to jog through some calculations without too much trouble. Just to remind you of these and give you a quick warm-up (you thought I'd forgotten the warm-up didn't you!), complete the following quick calculations:

EXERCISE 33

1. $10 \times 1000 =$ 4. $0.0125 \times 1000 =$
2. $0.004 \times 100 =$ 5. $50 \div 100 =$
3. $0.7 \div 10 =$

Got your breath back? Excellent. Check your answers on page 233 to see whether you are on the right tracks.

Okay, so you now know that a decimal point divides a number by 10. Moving the decimal point to the right increases the number by 10 times and to the left decreases the number by 10 times. Therefore if you divide 1 by 10 you will get 0.1. What you have done is divide the whole number 1 into 10 parts. Look at the box below that illustrates 1 divided into 10 parts.

1									
0.1	0.1	0.1	0.1	0.1	0.1	0.1	0.1	0.1	0.1

Another way of expressing 1 divided by 10 would be as a fraction and each part would be 1 tenth. If you took 3 parts of the box above what would you have? Hopefully you should have said 3 tenths. You can express this as ³⁄₁₀ (effectively this is 3 divided by 10) or if you actually do this calculation, that is, 3 divided by 10 you will get 0.3.

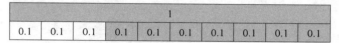

If you took 7 parts of the box above what would you have? Express this as a decimal and a fraction. Your answer should be ⁷⁄₁₀ or 0.7.

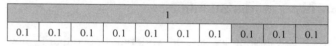

So to recap, we have whole numbers which are 'complete' numbers like 1, 2 and 3 and so on. If we have a part of a whole number, then we can express this as either a decimal or a fraction. Remember that a fraction literally means the top number divided by the bottom number, that is, ½ means take 1 and divide it into 2. What would ½ be expressed as a decimal? Can you see above how ½ would be 5 lots of 0.1s to give you 0.5?

Long division

I need to make a slight detour now to go through the skill of long division, which is useful for fractions and other questions where you need to divide. Long division is useful if you end up with a fraction as an answer, for example when you are multiplying fractions and need to work out what the decimal equivalent is of this or when a calculation requires you to divide numbers. Say you need to calculate how many millilitres a patient requires per hour if a 1000ml infusion is prescribed to infuse over 8 hours. Your calculation would be 1000 ÷ 8. If you do not know this answer from memory and you have no calculator, then you will have to do long division to work it out.

1000 ÷ 8 can be written as 8 ⟌ 1 0 0 0 by convention. The procedure basically requires you to consider how many 8s are in each number in turn. If the number is too small, then you move the number to the next one to 'make' a bigger number:

1. So we would ask how many 8s in 1 (remember that this number represents one thousand).
2. The answer is none so we move the 1 to the next number to 'make' 10 (again, remember that the 0 represents no hundreds) and ask the same thing.

$$\frac{0}{8\,\overline{)1\,_{10}0\,0}}$$

3. How many 8s in 10? There is one 8 in 10 with a remainder of 2. The 1 goes on top of the line and the remainder goes to the next number to 'make' 20.

$$\frac{0\ \ 1}{8\,\overline{)1\,_{10}\,_{20}0}}$$

4. How many 8s are there in 20? The answer is two 8s with a remainder of 4. Again the 2 goes on top and the 4 joins with the next zero to 'make' 40.

$$\frac{0\ \ 1\ \ 2}{8\,\overline{)1\,_{10}\,_{20}\,_{40}}}$$

5. How many 8s in 40? The answer is 5 with no remainder. The 5 goes on the line. The answer is the number on the line, which is 125.

$$\frac{0\ \ 1\ \ 2\ \ 5}{8\,\overline{)1\,_{10}\,_{20}\,_{40}}}$$

I appreciate that this seems a bit complicated. Once you try it a few times you will probably remember doing this at school and will begin to feel more familiar with the procedure.

You can use long division to work out the decimal equivalent to a fraction. For example, say you had finished multiplying fractions (we will cover how to do these shortly) and ended up with the answer $^{125}\!/_3$. This fraction $^{125}\!/_3$ means that you have 125 parts divided into 3. You can find the decimal equivalent by calculating $125 \div 3$. Long division is a way of calculating this answer. You set your calculation out as:

$$3\,\overline{)1\,2\,5}$$

The number inside the box is the number to be divided into parts and the number outside the number of parts you are going to divide it into.

Have a go at working this out on your before checking the answer and procedure below.

Answer

$$\frac{0\ \ 4\ \ 1\,.\,6\,6'}{3\,\overline{)1\,_{12}2\,5\,.\,_{20}2\,_{20}}}$$

Your procedure should have been something like this:

1. How many 3s are there in one, the first number? The answer is zero as the 3 is bigger.
2. You then move the 1 (which represents one hundred) to the next number to make 12 and ask how many 3s in 12.
3. The answer is 4 (3 x 4 = 12).
4. You place the 4 on top of the box and move onto the next number.
5. We then ask how many 3s in 5, which is 1 (1 x 3 = 3) with a remainder of 2.
6. We place the 1 on top of the box (make sure you've noted the decimal point) and move the 2 to the next number, which is a zero to make 20.
7. How many 3s in 20. This is 6 (3 x 6 = 18) with a remainder of 2 again.
8. This number now repeats.
9. The answer then is 41.666 recurring.

I will give you a few questions here to practise this. Make sure you have got the numbers in the right places, that is, the right one inside and outside your box.

EXERCISE 34

1. $250/9$
2. $3/8$
3. $1000/5$
4. $750 \div 5$
5. $675 \div 4$

(Answers: page 233)

Fractions

We need now to look at fractions in a bit more detail. You know that a fraction is a way of expressing a part of a whole number. Imagine you had a huge pizza that you had ordered from the takeaway just for you. Just as the pizza is delivered a friend turns up and invites themself to tea. You are a fair person so you divide the pizza into 2 equal parts (a). Then just as you are about to tuck in the doorbell rings and two more friends turn up. You now have to divide the pizza into 4 equal parts (b). Gritting your teeth as you see your slice of pizza get smaller and putting a smile on your face, you walk into the dining room only to hear the door bell go again as 4 more friends arrive (c). With a grimace, you valiantly divide the pizza up again. Finally, you sink into a chair with your even smaller slice. Raising the succulent pizza slice to your lips you are about to take a bite when 4 faces of more friends appear at the window. Throwing your slice back onto your plate in disgust and wishing you'd ordered the mega large pizza, you storm off into the kitchen to divide the pizza up again (d).

For each of the divisions above, work out what fraction of the pizza each person would be getting.

Answers

(a)   One pizza divided into 2 parts would give you a half or ½

(b)   One pizza now divided into 4 parts would give you a quarter or ¼

(c)   One pizza divided into 8 parts would give you an eighth or ⅛

(d)   Finally, one pizza divided into 12 (small!) parts would give you a twelfth or ¹⁄₁₂

The sharing of the one pizza can be illustrated like this (this is a new rectangular Italian pizza!).

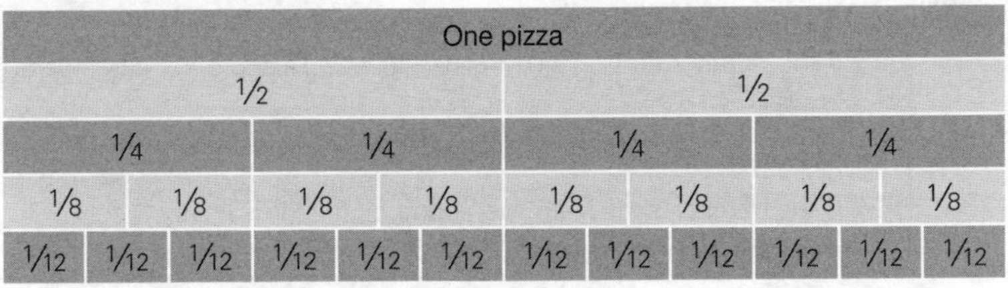

One pizza							
½				½			
¼		¼		¼		¼	
⅛	⅛	⅛	⅛	⅛	⅛	⅛	⅛
¹⁄₁₂	¹⁄₁₂	¹⁄₁₂	¹⁄₁₂	¹⁄₁₂	¹⁄₁₂	¹⁄₁₂	¹⁄₁₂	¹⁄₁₂	¹⁄₁₂	¹⁄₁₂	¹⁄₁₂

NB: For a full colour downloadable version see www.palgrave.com/nursinghealth/wright

So there you are, staring hungrily at the tiny slice of pizza you have, when the doorbell rings again. You groan in despair at the thought of more divisions. This time, though, it is the pizza delivery guy again with three more pizzas that one of your friends has ordered for you all. By this time your original pizza has been eaten so you now need to divide three pizzas into 12 equal parts. How would you do this? If you are stuck, look at the pizza above. If when you divided one pizza into 12 everyone got a twelfth, then this time everyone would get ¹⁄₁₂ of 3 pizzas or to put it another way ³⁄₁₂. Look again at the pizza above – how else could you express ³⁄₁₂? You should be able to see that ³⁄₁₂ is the same as ²⁄₈ and ¼.

Equivalent fractions

Fractions that have different numbers, but actually represent the same part of the whole are called equivalent fractions. You can create equivalent fractions by multiplying or dividing **both** the top and bottom number by the same number. So, for example, ½ is the same as ⁶/₁₂ (see above). In this case we have multiplied both top and bottom numbers by 6. What have you divided the top and bottom number by in the example above, when you had ³/₁₂, ²/₈, ¼? You should have seen that in ²/₈ you have divided both numbers by 2 to get ¼. With ³/₁₂, you have divided both top and bottom numbers by 3 to get ¼.

This principle is very useful when we have very large numbers in fractions to reduce them down to more manageable numbers. For example:

⁵⁰/₆₀ can have both 50 and 60 divided by 10 to give an equivalent fraction of ⁵/₆ (n.b. you should also notice that you are using your knowledge of dividing by 10s here by moving the decimal place one place to the left).

So basically, if you are faced with a horrendous looking fraction with huge numbers, look at the top and the bottom number to see what both could be divisible by. There are some tips to help you with this.

✔ Tips for Learning

- If the number ends in a 0, it is divisible by 10 and 5, for example 60 or 900
- If the number ends in a 0 or a 5, it is divisible by 5, for example 45 or 90
- If the number ends in an even number, it is divisible by 2, for example 12 or 212

Okay, some little brainteasers to see whether you have understood this so far. Complete the following questions then check your answers:

EXERCISE 35

1. Give two equivalent fractions for ⁴/₁₂.
2. Express ³/₄ in two different ways.
3. Express ½ in four different ways.
4. Give an equivalent fraction for ²⁵/₁₀₀.
5. Give an equivalent fraction for ⁴⁹/₈₄.

(Answers: page 233)

EXERCISE 36

1. What is the lowest equivalent fraction of $^{125}/_{500}$?
2. What is the lowest equivalent fraction of $^{500}/_{750}$?
3. Express $^2/_{10}$ as a decimal and give the lowest equivalent fraction.
4. Express 0.6 as a fraction and give another equivalent fraction for this.
5. What is the fraction equivalent of 0.75?

(Answers: page 234)

Multiplying fractions

First of all, let's take the three pizzas above which you needed to divide between 12 people. The calculation you could do for this would be $^1/_{12}$ as you want 12 pieces of pizza multiplied by 3 as this is the number of pizzas you have, therefore $^1/_{12}$ x 3. A way to ensure that you always do this type of calculation correctly is to think of the 3 as a fraction also. Obviously 3 is a whole number so you could represent it as a fraction as $^3/_1$. Your calculation would then be:

$$\frac{1 \times 3}{12 \times 1} = \frac{3}{12}$$

One of the reasons for making the 3 into a fraction is to ensure that you do not make the mistake of multiplying both the 1 and the 12 by 3 and ending up with $^3/_{36}$. If you think about this fraction, you should be able to see that it is smaller than $^1/_{12}$. You know that you should end up with a fraction that is bigger than $^1/_{12}$ as you are increasing it three times.

✔ **Tips for Learning**

The bigger the number on the bottom, the smaller the fraction. Thinking about your pizza that you had to keep dividing up, the more parts you had to divide it into, the smaller the pizza slice: $^1/_{12}$ is smaller than $^1/_2$. When you are multiplying fractions together, therefore, you multiply the top numbers together and then the bottom numbers. For example:

$$^1/_4 \times ^1/_2 = \frac{1 \times 1}{4 \times 2} = \frac{1}{8}$$

Try the following exercise to check you understand this (give your answers as the lowest equivalent fraction so you practise this as well!):

EXERCISE 37

1. $\frac{1}{3} \times \frac{1}{2} =$ 4. $\frac{3}{4} \times \frac{1}{2} =$
2. $\frac{1}{8} \times \frac{1}{2} =$ 5. $\frac{1}{8} \times \frac{4}{5} =$
3. $\frac{2}{5} \times \frac{1}{4} =$

(Answers: page 234)

Now back to the pizza. Imagine you had already divided your pizza into halves and then wanted to divide your half into four, your calculation would be ½ multiplied by ¼ as you want four parts of the half pizza. Another way to think of this is ½ divided by 4. It is difficult to express the calculation 1 divided by 2 divided by 4, so we use fractions. The calculation would be:

$$\frac{1 \times 1}{2 \times 4} = \frac{1}{8}$$

Can you see that multiplying by ¼ is the same as dividing by 4? Is ⅛ bigger or smaller than ¼ or ½? As the number on the bottom is bigger, we would expect the fraction to be smaller. I hope you would have expected it to be smaller anyway as you are dividing up your pizza half into smaller pieces!

Now, when we are multiplying numbers we are actually working out how many lots of a certain number we need. For example, 2 x 4 means two lots of four, which you all know gives a total of eight. When we are multiplying by fractions, we are doing a similar thing and are asking what is this fraction of this number. For example, ½ of 6 means that if I have six whole ones what would a half of this be? Hopefully you've all worked out that one half of 6 is 3. Try the questions below to see if you understand this:

EXERCISE 38

1. A half of 10 =   4. A third of 9 =
2. A quarter of 12 =   5. A tenth of 100 =
3. A fifth of 20 =

(Answers: page 234)

Can you see a pattern in how you worked out these answers? You should be able to see that you were actually dividing the number, so that a half of 10 is actually 10 divided by 2 and a tenth of 100 is 100 divided by 10.

Using mathematical notation, these questions would be written like this:

1. ½ x 10 = but what you are doing is 10 ÷ 2
2. ¼ x12 = 12 ÷ 4
3. ⅕ x 20 =20 ÷ 5
4. ⅓ x 9 = 9 ÷ 3
5. ⅒ x 100 = 100 ÷ 10

Now, being aware of the equivalent fractions and being able to reduce fractions down in a calculation can make life a lot easier for you, especially if you don't have a calculator handy. So we have said that you can reduce down fractions by dividing both top and bottom by the same number. You can extend this slightly if you are multiplying two fractions together. Consider the calculation below:

$$\frac{500}{4} \times \frac{20}{60}$$

You can reduce these numbers by simplifying each fraction separately, so dividing 500 and 4 by 4 gives you ¹²⁵⁄₁ and similarly, dividing 20 and 60 by 3 gives you ⅓:

$$\frac{125 \times 1}{3} = \frac{125 \times 1}{1 \times 3} = \frac{125}{3}$$

However, you can also reduce the size of the numbers by dividing **diagonally**. For the first calculation, this would be dividing either 500 and 60 by the same number or 20 and 4 by the same number. So you could divide 500 and 60 by 10 and 4 and 20 by 4 to give you:

$$\frac{50}{1} \times \frac{5}{6} = \frac{50 \times 5}{1 \times 6} = \frac{250}{6} = \frac{125}{3}$$

You will have the opportunity to practise these calculations in the end-of-session assessment. Before then, though, just to recap: you can simplify fractions by dividing either top and bottom, in the same fraction, by the same number, or by dividing numbers diagonally:

$$\updownarrow\frac{1000}{12} \underset{\nwarrow\nearrow}{\overset{\text{x}}{\searrow\swarrow}} \frac{15}{60}\updownarrow$$

Back to nursing

Some of you may be wondering what all this has got to do with nursing (apart from pizza slipping down just nicely after a long day!). You may remember the formula we use to work out drug dosages as being: what you want over what you have multiplied by what it's in. Sound familiar?

Okay, you have an ampoule of cyclizine (if you don't know what this is or what it is for, you need to BNF it!) which contains 100mg. If you had to divide this up into 4 equal parts how much would be in each part? Well done, 100mg divided by 4 would give you 25mg, which as you have worked out is a ¼.

What if, however, you needed to give 20mg? What fraction of the ampoule would you give now? What you need to do is work out the fraction. So you have 20mg out of 100mg. Before, when you had 25mg out of 100mg, you worked this out to be a quarter.

Although some of you probably knew this instinctively, what you are actually doing is $^{25}/_{100}$ and finding the equivalent by dividing top and bottom by 25 to get ¼. (To think of it another way, the ampoule contains 100 separate milligrams floating around. You want to take out 25 of those milligrams. You can express this as 25 out of 100 or 25 divided by 100.) So what fraction is 20mg of 100mg? $^{20}/_{100}$ is the equivalent of ⅕.

Okay, so you now know that you need to give one-fifth of the ampoule. This would still be tricky to work out without knowing how much liquid is in the ampoule in order to take out your fifth. If the ampoule contained 100mg in 1ml of cyclizine, how much would you draw up to give a fifth? Some of you may need a calculator to do this. Others may remember that ⅕ is equivalent to $^{2}/_{10}$, which is 0.2.

Therefore you would draw up 0.2ml (highly unlikely in reality unless you are doing paediatrics). What if the cyclizine was 100mg in 2ml? Remember, you know that you want a fifth of the ampoule. So imagine you are dividing the ampoule into 5 parts and want 2 parts of this. In other words ⅕ multiplied by 2, which gives you 0.4ml.

To put this all together, what you are doing when you use the formula is finding out the fraction that you want of the ampoule (what you want divided by what you have) then working out what fraction of liquid this would be (multiplied by what it's in).

Just to check you have understood this, I will give you another example. You want 75mg of a drug. The ampoules you have contain 250mg the drug in 2ml. You want to find out the fraction that 75 is of 250 and then work out what fraction of liquid this would give you. Your calculation should therefore be 75 divided by 250 to give you your fraction and then multiply this by 2 to work out how much liquid to draw up. So this is $^{75}/_{250}$ x 2. How much of the drug would you draw up? Check your answer.

Worked example and answer

You require 75mg of the drug and have 250mg/2ml ampoules:

$$\frac{75 \times 2}{250 \times 1} = \frac{150}{250} = \frac{15}{25} = \frac{3}{5} = 0.6\text{ml}$$

So far we have covered the arithmetic that you will need to help you in nursing. At times, however, you may be asked to do a general numeracy test which can include calculations involving fractions and which we haven't covered here yet. These calculations are adding fractions together and dividing by fractions. Very rarely, if ever, would you have to do these types of calculations in clinical practice but you will need to understand the principles of how these calculations work for nursing. Let's take division of fractions first as we have already briefly mentioned this in relation to pizzas.

Division of fractions

It is important to remember what a fraction represents. A fraction means a part of a whole and is basically stating that you have divided the whole into a certain number of parts. So ½ is one whole one divided into two parts and ⅜ is a whole one divided into eight parts and three of those eight parts. We can represent these fractions as diagrams, which makes them easier to visualise:

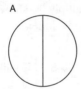
A

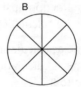
B

Each section here represents 1/2   Each section here represents 1/8
                                         so three sections would be 3/8

Now if we needed to work out 12 divided by 2, we are really asking how many 2s are there in 12 or how many 2s 'fit' into 12. The answer here is that you can fit six 2s into the number 12. Now when we want to work out 6 divided by ½ we are actually asking how many halves will 'fit' into six. This can be visualised as each of the six whole ones each being divided in half:

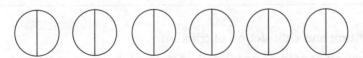

If you count the number of pieces we now have you should get the answer of 12. So:

$6 \div \frac{1}{2} = 12$

To give another example: imagine you need to work out ¼ divided ⅛. Remember that we are trying to work out how many eighths can be fitted into ¼. Look at the diagrams below:

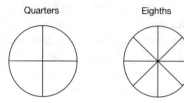

Quarters   Eighths

Can you see how many of the eighths would fit into one quarter just by looking? Hopefully you can see that two eighths will fit into one quarter so the calculation and answer is:

¼ ÷ ⅛ = 2

It would be a very time consuming if we had to keep drawing circles to work out any division involving fractions, but thankfully there is an easy way of calculating these problems. Basically, if you want to divide by a fraction you turn the fraction upside down and multiply. To show you how this works, I will use the calculations we have already done:

6 ÷ ½ is the same as calculating 6 x ²/₁ or just 6 x 2

¼ ÷ ⅛ is the same as calculating ¼ x ⁸/₁ or just ¼ x 8. This will give ⁸/₄ which can be simplified to 2.

EXERCISE 39

1. ¼ ÷ ⅙ =

2. 2 ÷ ⅕ =

3. ⅓ ÷ ⅙ =

4. 4 ÷ ⅛ =

5. ⅖ ÷ ¹/₁₀ =

(Answers: page 234)

Addition and subtraction of fractions

When you are adding or subtracting fractions you are basically working out a total of the fractions put together or what is left when one is taken away from the other. To give some everyday examples you will be familiar with, taking ½ away from a whole one, for example if you've eaten half of a cake knowing how much is left and being able to work out that two halves of the cake make a whole cake. In mathematical notation this can be written as $1 - \frac{1}{2}$ and $\frac{1}{2} + \frac{1}{2}$.

Now when the fractions being added are from the same portions, that is, as above, both are halves represented by the bottom number (known as the denominator) as 2, then you can do a straightforward addition or subtraction sum. However, when the fractions are different, for example you may be adding together fifths and thirds, you cannot just add them, but must work out, for each fraction, equivalent fractions that have the same denominator (bottom number). For example, you may need to convert both fractions into twelfths by working out the number of twelfths that are in each of the fractions you need to add up. This is similar to having to convert euros to pounds before you can work out the total amount of money you have.

I appreciate that this sounds complicated and it can cause a lot of confusion. However, if you just remember that you must add and subtract like with like when dealing with fractions, follow the steps below and practise and practise, you will soon be confident with this.

Example

$\frac{1}{4} + \frac{1}{4} =$

First you need to recognise that the denominators are the same so the fractions are the same type. Therefore you can just add these numbers as usual by adding the top number together and keeping the same bottom number:

$$\frac{1}{4} + \frac{1}{4} \longrightarrow \frac{= 2}{= 4} \text{ reduce down to equivalent fractions to get } \frac{1}{2}$$

Guide

1. Consider the bottom number of each fraction to see if they are in the same 'family', that is, same denominator
2. If they are, add the top numbers together and keep the bottom number the same
3. Reduce fraction to the smallest equivalent fraction by dividing the top and bottom numbers by the same number

Example

$\frac{1}{2} + \frac{1}{4} =$

Here you need to recognise that the fractions are different (the denominators, that is, bottom numbers, are different). One fraction is a half and the other is a quarter. In this example you need to find a common fraction for them both. To do this, you find the smallest number that both of the fractions denominators can go into. In this example I would chose the number 4. Now I need to work out what is ½ in quarters so both fractions are from the same 'family'. You may already know that ½ is the same as ²⁄₄, but, if not, you can work this out as you do your sum:

1. Consider the bottom number of each fraction to see if they are in the same 'family', that is, same denominator:

    ½ + ¼ = denominators are different

2. If they are different, then find a common number that both of the fractions denominators will go into:

    Both numbers will go into 4

3. Make this number the denominator for both fractions:

    $$\frac{1}{2} + \frac{1}{4} = \frac{\qquad}{4}$$

4. Now you need to work out the fractions converted to the common denominator:

    Stage 1

    ½ + ¼ = $\frac{2 +}{4}$

    2 into 4 = 2

    2 x 1 = 2

    Stage 2

    ½ + ¼ = $\frac{2 + 1}{4}$

    4 into 4 = 1

    1 x 1 = 1

5. Add the top numbers together:

    $$\frac{2 + 1}{4} = \frac{3}{4}$$

6. Reduce fraction to lowest equivalent fraction.

For subtracting fractions, you do exactly the same processes until you get to point 5 above. For addition, you add these numbers together. For subtraction, you take them away.

EXERCISE 40

1. $\frac{1}{2} + \frac{1}{3} =$
2. $\frac{3}{4} + \frac{1}{2} =$
3. $\frac{3}{5} - \frac{1}{5} =$

4. $\frac{1}{8} + \frac{1}{2} =$
5. $\frac{2}{5} - \frac{3}{8} =$

(Answers: page 234)

✔ Tips for Learning

If you cannot think of a number, multiply both of the denominator numbers together.

Summary

To recap. In this session you have looked at the relationship between fractions and decimals and should now know how to convert between the two. You have also looked at fractions; how to reduce down and how to multiply fractions. Finally, we have related this back to nursing for you to see how all of these skills are important to be able to perform drug calculations and to understand what you are doing and make sense of your answers. As a little extra we have put in division, subtraction and addition of fractions so you are aware of how to do these calculations for numeracy tests.

I hope you have found this session helpful. Now have a go at the assessment for this session:

Assessment Session Two

1. Express 0.5 as a fraction

2. Express $\frac{1}{8}$ as a decimal

3. $\frac{1}{10} \times 1000 =$

4. $\dfrac{1000}{8} \times \dfrac{20}{60} =$

5. $\frac{20}{50} \times 2 =$

6. $\frac{1}{4} \div \frac{1}{8} =$

7. $\frac{1}{5} + \frac{2}{3} =$

8. $\frac{1}{2} - \frac{1}{8} =$

9. You need to administer 5mg of a drug from an ampoule of strength 20mg/2ml. How many millilitres would you need to administer?

10. You need to give 60mg of a drug. The elixir available for this drug contains 15mg/2ml. How many millilitres do you need to administer?

(Answers: page 235)

● Session Three – How Supple Are You?

Welcome to the third session in your maths exercise programme. Congratulations to those that have worked their way doggedly through sessions one and two. I hope you are beginning to reap the benefits of your hard work!

In this session we are going to cover percentages. To do this, you will need to apply many of the principles that you have covered in the previous sessions. You will therefore need to 'stretch, bend and reach' further with the mathematical knowledge you have gained so far and show how supple you have become with your workouts to date.

Percentages

Some of you may be familiar with the term 'per cent', which you will sometimes see written as 'percent' as well as the symbol %. Per means 'for each' and 'cent' means a 'hundred' (n.b. think of century). So per cent basically means 'for each hundred'. Translating literally then, if you had 20%, this means 20 for each hundred and 3% means 3 for each hundred. If I gave you 100 sweets and you ate 28 of these, what percentage have you eaten? Hopefully you would have worked out that you would have eaten 28%. This is quite easy to see when your quantity is 100. Look at the following questions and express each of the pieces of information as a percentage:

EXERCISE 41

1. 15g out of 100g
2. 75ml out of 100ml
3. 40 sweets out of 100 sweets
4. 25 donkeys out of 100 donkeys
5. 10mcg out of 100mcg

(Answers: page 235)

Make sure you are clear about this before moving on.

Percentages as fractions

Another way of expressing a percentage is to write it as a fraction. So your whole part is the 100 and the 'part' of this is the number expressed. With this fraction, you are always expressing the fraction as hundredths. For example, 30% would be 30 out of 100 which would be expressed as a fraction as $\frac{30}{100}$. The astute among you will have noticed already that you can reduce this fraction down to $\frac{3}{10}$ by dividing both the top and bottom number by 10. Now go back to the above questions and express these as fractions. Try to reduce your answer as the lowest equivalent fraction. Check your answers to this exercise:

1. 15g out of 100g = 15% = $\frac{15}{100}$ = $\frac{3}{20}$ (dividing top and bottom by 5)
2. 75ml out of 100ml = 75% = $\frac{75}{100}$ = $\frac{3}{4}$ (dividing top and bottom by 25)
3. 40 sweets out of 100 sweets = 40% = $\frac{40}{100}$ = $\frac{2}{5}$ (dividing top and bottom by 20)
4. 25 donkeys out of 100 donkeys = 25% = $\frac{25}{100}$ = $\frac{1}{4}$ (dividing top and bottom by 25)
5. 10mcg out of 100mcg = 10% = $\frac{10}{100}$ = $\frac{1}{10}$ (dividing top and bottom by 10)

Okay, hopefully this has been quite straightforward for most of you and you can see that, for example, when you get 75 questions right out of a possible 100, this is the same as saying that you got 75% right or $\frac{3}{4}$ of the questions right. How then would you work out a percentage of a number that is different from 100? For example what is 75% of 400?

You could actually do this several ways:

1.   Method 1 – Thinking logically
     You know 75% means 75 out of every hundred. So if you have 400, then you have 75 for each of the 100s. As there are 4 lots of 100 then you have 4 lots of 75. The calculation is 75 x 4, which is 300. 75% of 400 is therefore 300.

2.   Method 2 – Using a calculation
     You know that 75% can also be expressed as $^{75}/_{100}$, which is the same as saying you want ¾ of 400 (reducing down to the smallest equivalent fraction). Using your knowledge of multiplying with fractions, you want ¾ x 400 = 300.

3.   Method 3 – Using your knowledge of equivalent fractions
     $^{75}/_{100}$ is the same as $^{150}/_{200}$, which is the same as $^{300}/_{400}$. Therefore the answer is 300.

Using the methods in this example work out 40% of 250. Check your answer once you have done this to ensure you understand it. I have given the answers using all three ways you could do this, but you need only use one way (unless you want to really stretch yourself in which case by all means use all three ways).

Answer

1.   Method 1

Logically. If you have 40 out of every hundred, you will also have 20 out of every 50. So I have 2 lots of 100s and 1 lot of 50:

40 in 100
40 in 100
20 in 50
= 40 + 40 + 20
= 100

2.   Method 2
Calculating:

$^{40}/_{100}$ x 250
= $^{2}/_{5}$ x 250
= 100

3.   Method 3
Equivalents:

$^{40}/_{100} = ^{80}/_{200} = ^{100}/_{250}$

Once you have found the way that suits you best (most of you will probably chose the calculation method, which is the simplest way especially when the numbers get more complex), complete the following exercise then check your answers:

EXERCISE 42

Work out the following values:
1. 10% of 164
2. 5% of 1000
3. 72% of 36
4. 2% of 48
5. 0.9% of 1000

(Answers: page 235)

? Maths Explained

The word 'of' in mathematical terms is the same as multiplying. So that 1/2 of 50 is the same as 1/2 x 50.

If you found these too easy, try these 'bonus' questions:

EXERCISE 43

If the percentage of solute in an infusion is always expressed as grams, that is, 5% = 5 grams in 100ml, answer the following:

1. How many grams of glucose in 1000ml infusion bag of 5% glucose?
2. How many grams of sodium chloride in 1000ml 0.9% sodium chloride infusion bag?

(Answers: page 235)

Percentages as decimals

More suppleness required now. If you can express percentages as fractions, then it stands to reason that you can also express them as decimals. So 10% is $^{10}/_{100}$, which is 10 divided by 100 and is 0.1 (remembering that you move the decimal point two places to the left). You could also reduce $^{10}/_{100}$ to the equivalent fraction of $^1/_{10}$ and know that this is 0.1 expressed as a decimal.

Example

What is 70% expressed as a decimal?

$70\% = {}^{70}/_{100} = {}^7/_{10} = 0.7$

Being able to recognise fractions as decimals and percentages can be useful when you are doing calculations, but will also help you to understand what it is you are doing. Use the following exercise to test your recognition skills!

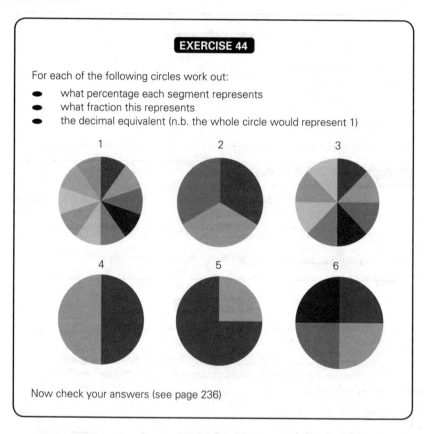

EXERCISE 44

For each of the following circles work out:

- what percentage each segment represents
- what fraction this represents
- the decimal equivalent (n.b. the whole circle would represent 1)

1   2   3

4   5   6

Now check your answers (see page 236)

Finding percentages

What if you got 15 questions right in a quiz out of a possible 20? How would you work out what percentage of questions you have got right? First, what you need to do is express this as a fraction. So you have 15 out of 20, which is $^{15}/_{20}$. Now you can either use your knowledge to work out that $^{15}/_{20}$ is the same as $^{75}/_{100}$ (multiplying both top and bottom by 5), which is therefore 75%, or work out what fraction $^{15}/_{20}$ is of 100:

$$\frac{15}{20} \times 100 = \frac{3}{4} \times 100 = 75\%$$

Okay, now try this example:

Example

If you have 50g glucose and you dissolved this into 1000ml of water, what percentage glucose would you have? (Don't be put off by the language here.)

Firstly, you have 50 out of 1000. The fraction therefore is $^{50}/_{1000}$. You then need to work out what fraction $^{50}/_{1000}$ is of 100:

$$\frac{50}{1000} \times 100 = \frac{50}{10} \times 1 = 5\%$$

Have a go at some more examples to check you have fully understood this.

EXERCISE 45

1. You get 37 questions right out of a possible 50. What percentage have you got right?

2. Wayne Rooney scores 15 goals out of a possible 184 shots. What percentage does he score (you can tell I'm not a Manchester United fan!)?

3. A pair of trousers has been reduced from £40 to £28. What is the percentage reduction (n.b. how many pounds have they been reduced by)?

4. 42 student nurses get over 65% in a maths test. There are 60 students in the group. What percentage gets over 65%?

5. You have £50 in your purse when you go out shopping. When you get back home you have only got £4 left. What percentage of your money have you spent?

(Answers: page 236)

If this is a bit overwhelming and you don't know where to start, I have given you the first step here:

1. You get 37 questions right out of a possible 50. What percentage have you got right? $^{37}/_{50} \times 100$

2. Wayne Rooney scores 15 goals out of a possible 184 shots. What percentage does he score? $^{15}/_{184} \times 100$

3. A pair of trousers has been reduced from £40 to £28. What is the percentage reduction (n.b. how many pounds have they been reduced by)? Trousers reduced by £12. Therefore $^{12}/_{40} \times 100$

4. 42 student nurses get over 65% in a maths test. There are 60 students in the group. What percentage gets over 65%? $^{42}/_{60} \times 100$

5. You have £50 in your purse when you go out shopping. When you get back home you have only got £4 left. What percentage of your money have you spent? Money spent is 50 – 4 = 46. $^{46}/_{50} \times 100$

Percentage increases and decreases

There is just one other last thing which is useful for you to know about percentages and which is useful for nursing as well as everyday life and that is working out the percentage increase and decrease to a value (this is especially vital when comparing those bargains in the sales!).

Okay, so you are walking past a shop window and it states 20% reduction on all marked prices. You quite fancy this jumper that is marked as £30. How would you work out the sale price? There are two steps:

1. Work out 20% of £30
2. Take this amount from £30

So for this example:

1. 20% of £30 would be $^{20}/_{100}$ x 30 = £6
2. £30 – £6 = £24

You would apply the same principles if you want to work out an increase, except that in step two you would **add** this amount to your original amount:

1. Work out percentage increase
2. Add this amount to your original

So if the jumper had been increased in price by 20%, this would be £36.

Now putting this together, what if your jumper was £22 reduced from £30? How would you work out the percentage reduction on the jumper? Again there are two steps:

1. Work out the amount of discount: here it would be £30 – £22 = £8
2. Work out what percentage this is of the original value: $^{8}/_{30}$ x 100 = 26.7%

Now try these quick examples.

EXERCISE 46

1. A patient has reduced their weight from 72kg to 68kg. What percentage decrease is this?
2. A patient has had 800ml of a 1000ml infusion. What percentage infusion have they had?
3. After an intensive exercise programme, a patient's heart rate has decreased by 15%. If it was 110 bpm (beats per minute) before the programme started, what is it now?

4. Your patient's body mass index (BMI) has increased by 30% from 20. What is their present BMI?
5. Your patient who has COPD (chronic obstructive pulmonary disease) is thrilled that they are now able to walk 25% further than 4 weeks ago when they could only walk 40m. How far can your patient now walk?

(Answers: page 236)

If you have got this far and worked through all the exercises, then you must be a very toned and supple mathematician by now! Well done. I hope you have found this session useful and continue practising every time you see figures expressed in percentages … you may just realise that the bargain you've spotted is not quite such as good a bargain as you thought!

Try the assessment for session three before moving on to the next session.

Assessment Session Three

1. Complete the following table:

Fractions	Decimals	Percentages
		50
	0.6	
¼		
		75%
⅕		

2. 15 out of 25 patients on your ward are receiving Intravenous antibiotics (IVAB). What percentage of patients on your ward are receiving IVAB?

3. Express $^{25}/_{125}$ as a percentage.

4. Express 25% as a decimal.

5. Through effective medicines management, you manage to reduce your patient's morning medication from 20 tablets to 15 tablets. What percentage have your reduced your patient's morning tablets by?

6. How many grams of glucose are dissolved in a 5% 1000ml infusion bag?

7. Your patient's medication dose needs to be increased by 10%. Currently the dose is 20mg. What will the new dose be?

8. What is 25% of 1000?

9. Your patient has received 200ml of a 500ml infusion before it is discontinued. What percentage of the infusion has the patient received?

10. The emergency admission numbers in your hospital have reduced from 1250 to 1200 for this month. The target for the hospital is to reduce emergency admissions by 5%. Has your hospital met this target?

(Answers: page 236)

Session Four – Through the Pain Barrier!

Welcome to the fourth session in your maths exercise programme. Some of you may be feeling a bit tired by now and have been thinking about giving it all up and hoping you won't have to do any drug calculations in practice (unlikely!). Don't give up. If you stay with it and run through the pain barrier, before you know it, you'll be cruising along happily and will be tackling any drug calculation that comes your way with ease …

Right onwards … so far we have covered several different ways of expressing when we have some part of a whole item. This item could be anything from an ampoule of medication to a pizza! A part of a whole can be expressed as:

- A decimal
- A fraction
- A percentage

How would you express a half of a pizza in each of these three ways? Check your answer:

A half can be expressed as:

- A decimal = 0.5
- A fraction = ½
- A percentage = 50%

Ratios

There is one final way that parts can be expressed which is useful for nursing and that is as **ratios.** To understand ratios, we first need to recap on fractions. Remember that a fraction consists of a bottom number that tells you how many parts there are altogether in the whole one, for example if you divided your pizza into 2 you would have 2 parts of pizza. Your top number is the number of parts you have taken from the whole one. So if you ate 1 piece, you would have eaten 1 part of the whole (2) = ½.

You can find equivalent fractions by multiplying or dividing the top and bottom number by the same amount. An equivalent fraction to ½ = $^{25}/_{50}$ (multiplying top and bottom numbers by 25).

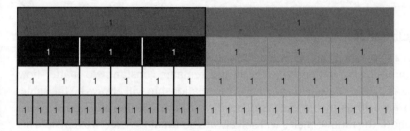

Look at the diagram above. Even though each row has been divided into more and more pieces, the black outlined sections on the left still represent ½. The bottom row of this section has 12 pieces out of a possible 24 so can be expressed as $^{12}/_{24}$. Hopefully this diagram will help you to see that this is still ½.

Another way you could express this is to say that there are 12 parts compared to the whole 24. You could write this as 12:24. This is a ratio and allows you to compare the part you have to the whole amount. What would the ratio of the white section above be to the whole section? There are 6 pieces to a total of 12 so it would be 6:12. What about the black section? This is 3 parts of a total of 6 so would be 3:6.

Ratios are helpful in comparing one part with another. These parts can be drugs dissolved into a whole solution, pepperoni slices per pizza or males to female on a caseload. For example, a ratio of 3:4 dogs to cats at a rescue centre is basically saying that for every 3 cats at the centre there will always be 4 dogs. Another way of saying this is ¾ of all the cats and dogs (the whole one) will be cats. Try these questions below to check your understanding of this. Check your answers once you have done this.

EXERCISE 47

1. The ratio of olives to each pizza from Planet Zog's pizzeria is always 4:1. If I ordered a pizza how many olives would I get?
2. The ratio of male to female students in a nursing cohort is 1:10. If a cohort has 10 females how many will be male? Express the number of males as a fraction.
3. The ratio of adrenaline (g) to solution (ml) is 1:1000. How many grams of adrenaline in 1000ml? Express the amount of adrenaline as a fraction of the solution.

(Answers: page 237)

Relationships

An important thing to remember about ratios is that because they are expressing a relationship, this always remains constant. No matter how many pizzas or students you have, the relationship will always be the same. So even if, as in the exercise above, you have 250 female students in a cohort, the ratio to males will still always be 1 male to every 10 female. This means that you can use ratios to work out the amount of one variable if you know the first variable. For example, in the questions above you knew that the ratio of olives to pizza was 4:1 and that you had 1 pizza. This means that you can work out that you would get 4 olives. This is obviously an easy example. What if you were having a big party and ordered 25 pizzas, how many olives would you have in total then? Because you know that the ratio is 4:1 you would get 25 lots of 4 olives, which is 25 multiplied by 4 to get 100 olives. See if you follow the next examples:

The ratio of sweets eaten by Colm compared to Millish is 3:2:

1. If Colm eats 3 sweets, how many will Millish eat?

	Colm	Millish
Ratio	3	2

The ratio is 3:2, so if Colm has 3, Millish will eat 2

2. If Colm eats 6 sweets, how many will Millish eat?

	Colm		Millish
Ratio	3	x2	2
Sweets	6 ↓		? ↓

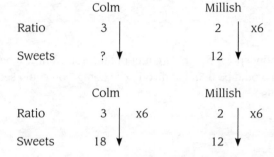

	Colm		Millish	
Ratio	3	x2	2	x2
Sweets	6		4	

The relationship stays constant between Colm and Millish's sweet eating capabilities. Therefore if Colm eats 6, this is twice the ratio amount. As the ratio is always constant, we double Millish's ratio to get 4 sweets.

3.   If Millish eats 12 sweets, how many will Colm eat?

	Colm		Millish	
Ratio	3		2	x6
Sweets	?		12	

	Colm		Millish	
Ratio	3	x6	2	x6
Sweets	18		12	

Remembering that as the relationship remains constant, whatever happens to one side of the ratio must also happen to the other. Here Millish has eaten 12, which is 6 times the ratio. Colm will therefore also eat 6 times as many sweets, which is 6 x 3 = 18.

Some of you may have noticed that this is the same principle as equivalent fractions where $\frac{3}{8} = \frac{6}{16} = \frac{16}{32}$. Whatever you do to the top number, you must do to the bottom number. Using these principles, 3:4 is the same as:

12:15 = 30:40 = 75:100 = 6:8

See if you can now apply these principles to the following questions and check you answers.

EXERCISE 48

1.   Jack always gets $\frac{1}{2}$ of his exam questions right. What ratio does Jack get right?
2.   Express $\frac{4}{24}$ as the smallest ratio.
3.   You have 1000:1000 adrenaline ampoules (mg/ml). If you gave 1ml, how many milligrams of adrenaline would you have administered?

(Answers: page 237)

More advanced

You can actually use the principles of ratios to work out drug dosages. The formula *'what you want over what you have multiplied by what it's in'* is really what you are doing when you find out what one side of the ratio has been multiplied or divided by, and then doing the same to the other side. Say you wanted to give 20mg cyclizine to a patient. The ampoules on the ward are 100mg in 2ml. The ratio here is 100mg:2ml. Equivalent ratios are:

100mg:2ml
dividing both sides by 2 gives
50mg:1ml
dividing both sides by 2 gives
25mg:0.5ml

As an estimate, you now know that the amount of fluid you want will be less than 0.5ml as 25mg would be 0.5ml and you need 20mg. You could set your problem out like this:

100mg:2ml
20mg:?

What you are asking yourself is: what has happened to the 100mg to give 20mg? Once you know this, you need only do the same to the other side of the ratio. The 100mg has been divided by 5 to give 20mg or has been multiplied by a fifth. This is:

$\frac{20}{100}$. You then multiply 2 by $\frac{20}{100}$ or a fifth or alternatively you could just divide 2ml by five. This gives you 0.4ml.
(20 = what you want, 100 = what you have, 2 = what it's in)

Obviously the formula is a lot simpler for some people, but it is useful sometimes to be able to think what it is you are actually doing when you use the formulas.

Summary

That is all I think you will need to know about ratios. If you remember that ratios express a relationship that is constant and that whatever you do to one side you must do to the other, this will help you to understand drugs expressed as ratios, such as adrenaline and heparin.

Check you understand what we have covered in this session by completing the assessment for session four before moving on to the final session.

Assessment Session Four

1. The ratio of chocolate to staff in your team is always 5:2. If there are 2 staff on duty today, how many chocolates will they get?

2. The ratio of community matrons to patients should be 1:50. How many patients should one community matron case manage?

3. A patient is assessed as needing the assistance of 2 staff for transferring from bed to chair. Express this as a ratio of staff to patient.

4. The ratio of qualified staff to patients on a unit must be 2:12. You have 36 patients on your unit. How many staff do you require?

5. The strength of an adrenaline ampoule is 1:1000 (g:ml). If you administer 3 ampoules of this adrenaline, how many milligrams have you administered? (1g = 1000mg)

6. The ratio of drug to volume in an elixir is 10mg:2ml. You need to administer 30mg. How many millilitres would this be?

7. The dose of an adrenaline ampoule is 1:1000 (g:ml). How many milligrams in 1ml? (Note that I am asking for your answer to be in milligrams – n.b. 1g = 1000mg.)

8. A drug dose must always be diluted to give a ratio of 1:10 (mg:ml). The drug dose is 10mg. How many millilitres do you need to dilute this with?

9. The adrenaline ampoule strength is 1:100 (g:ml). Express this ratio in milligrams (n.b. 1g = 1000mg).

10. Express the adrenaline 1:1000 (g:ml) strength in the ratio of milligrams to millilitres.

(Answers: page 237)

● Session Five – Running the 5K Maths Challenge!

Welcome to the final session in this maths series. If you have completed all the exercises so far, then you should be feeling pretty good about your chances in this 5K run! Hopefully you'll have done your warm-ups and are now confidently jogging on the spot ready for the starting gun to go so you can demonstrate what you can do.

The 5K Maths Challenge will consist of 12 laps that you will need to complete in order to finish the run. The run has been devised so you can test your understanding of the maths concepts we have covered to date and to give you the chance to apply these to nursing practice. Good luck!

'On your marks,'
'Get set,'
'GO!'

Lap 1

Mrs Jones is in pain. Her pain score is 8 (on a scale of 0–10, where 0 = no pain). On her medicine chart is the following information:

morphine 20mg IM
diclofenac 50mg PO
paracetamol 1g PO

None of the above has been administered in the last 6 hours.
You decide to administer the morphine.
The information on the ampoule is 50mg/2ml.

1. How many millilitres from this morphine ampoule would you administer?

Lap 2

You go back to Mrs Jones 4 hours later and her pain score is now 4 using the same scale. She has received no other analgesia since you last gave her the morphine.

You decide to administer both the diclofenac and the paracetamol.
When you go the drug trolley, the only tablets available for diclofenac are 25mg and for the paracetamol 500mg.

How many tablets would you give:
1. Of the diclofenac?
2. Of the paracetamol?

Lap 3

Sunita has been prescribed 15 000 units of heparin over 24 hours IV. Heparin needs to be administered in an infusion of sodium chloride 0.9% in a 50ml syringe and administered via a syringe pump. The ampoules in stock contain 25 000 units/ml.

1. How many millilitres of the ampoule would you draw up?

Lap 4

You have drawn up the volume of heparin required (from the answer to Lap 3) and have added this to your 50ml syringe. You then draw up enough sodium chloride to make the infusion amount 50ml.

1. How many millilitres of sodium chloride would you need to draw up to make up the total volume to 50ml in the syringe? (Hint: this is the total volume of 50ml minus the volume you calculated for Lap 3.)

Lap 5

Jessica requires 20mg oramorph. The oramorph bottle you have in stock contains an oramorph solution of 10mg /5ml.

1. How many millilitres would you administer for Jessica?

Lap 6

Jessica's pain has not been well controlled on the 20mg dose of oramorph so it is increased by 50%.

1. What dose of oramorph is Jessica now on?

Lap 7

You visit Mr Chandra at home who is concerned about his medication. He has been told that he should take 0.25mg of digoxin daily, but has been given tablets that are 125mcg. It says on the digoxin bottle to take 4 tablets daily. Mr Chandra was unsure about this so decided to wait until you visited to ask you!

1. How many tablets should Mr Chandra take to give a dose of 250mcg?
2. What dose would taking 4 tablets from this bottle give?

Lap 8

Look at the following intravenous fluid medicine administration chart.

Sunnydene and Reynold NHS Trust

Intravenous medicine administration chart

Name: Fred Kumar   **Hospital Number:** 0789655   **Consultant:** Rogers

Date of Birth: 1/9/1952   **Ward:** Oak

Date prescribed	Solution	Volume	Duration of infusion	Date to be given	Prescriber's signature
1/2/2011	5% glucose	1000ml	8 hours	1/2/2011	R Dickenson

1. If you were setting up the 5% glucose infusion for Fred with a crystalloid giving set (20 drops/ml), calculate how many drips per minute you would set the infusion up for. NB: Use the formula:

$$\frac{\text{volume to be administered}}{\text{duration (in hours)}} \times \frac{\text{drop/ml}}{60} = \text{drips per minute}$$

Lap 9

Looking again at Fred's intravenous medicine administration chart above, how many grams of glucose would Fred be given at the end of his 8-hour glucose infusion?

Lap 10

Look at Fred's intravenous medicine administration chart above again and calculate the rate per hour in millilitres to infuse the glucose via a volu-metric pump.

Lap 11

There are 30 patients on Baldrick ward: 20% of these patients have pressure sores, 80% have IVs running and 50% have been prescribed laxatives.

Work out the number of patients:
1. With pressure sores
2. Who have IVs
3. Who have been prescribed laxatives

Lap 12

Baldrick ward also has a ratio of staff to patients on an early shift of 1:6. Using the information in Lap 11, work out how many staff work on an early shift.

(Answers: page 237)

If you have managed to get all these questions right then come forward and receive your 5K maths finisher's medal. Congratulations.

5 How much have I learnt? A chance to evaluate your learning

66 200 questions to assess your learning, help you revise and prepare you for written drug calculation assessments 99

This chapter contains ten assessments for you to evaluate your learning and prepare for any written drug tests you may be required to sit. I have based each assessment on specific areas of drug calculations which I hope will help you to focus on the areas of calculations relevant to you. The first six assessments are based on the calculations covered in Chapters 1–3 (two assessments for each chapter). These are very useful to check your understanding of calculations covered in those chapters and for further revision.

I have also included an assessment that specifically covers calculations found in adult nursing and one that contains calculations specific to children's nursing. Finally, I am aware of the differences in calculations required between acute nursing and community nursing so have also included two separate assessments for these two areas of practice. There is, of course, nothing stopping you from doing all of these assessments!

Warning!
Please remember that being able to answer the written questions does not mean that you will be completely competent in solving drug calculations in your practice area. As always, I advise that you find the time to practise drug calculations as part of your medicine administration in the clinical context so that you can apply and make sense of the skills you have learnt in this book.

● Assessment 1 – Calculating and understanding simple medicine dosages

(based on Chapter 1)

1. Your patient has been prescribed 1.2g benzylpenicillin. The vials available contain 0.6g. How many vials do you need to administer to give this dose?

2. You need to administer 500mg amoxicillin. The tablets available are 250mg. How many tablets do you need to administer to give this dose?

3. The prescription for digoxin for your patient is 0.25mg. The tablets available are 125mcg. How many tablets do you need to administer?

4. A baby you are caring for has been prescribed 7.5mg/kg clarithromycin. The baby weighs 5.4kg. How many milligrams of clarithromycin does the baby require?

5. Your patient has been prescribed 300mg aminophylline. The tablets available are 100mg tablets. How many tablets do you need to administer?

6. Your patient has been prescribed amoxicillin 375mg in three divided doses. How many milligrams does your patient require for each dose?

7. A child has been prescribed 2mg/kg gentamicin every 12 hours. What dose does the child require if they weigh 19kg?

8. The nurse has prescribed your patient 30mg diazepam in three divided doses. The tablets available are 5mg. How many tablets would you administer for each dose?

9. You need to administer 0.45g dipyridamole in three divided doses to your patient. There are two tablet strengths available: 100mg and 50mg. How many of the tablets would you administer to your patient for each dose?

10. How many milligrams of adrenaline are there in a 1ml ampoule of adrenaline 1:1000?

Use the following medicine chart and available drug strengths to calculate questions 11–13:

Sunnydene and Reynold NHS Trust

Name: Davy Thomlinson   **Hospital Number:** 0114567

Weight: 60kg   **Height:** 155cm

REGULAR PRESCRIPTIONS

Year 2011	Date & Month 1st February			Date Time												
Drug Gentamicin				07.00												
				09.00												
Dose 2mg/kg	Route IM	Start date 1/2/11	Valid period 14 days	12.00												
				14.00												
Signature R Dickinson		Dispensed 1/2/11		18.00												
				22.00												
Additional comments																
Drug Morphine sulphate				07.00												
				09.00												
Dose 60mg	Route IM	Start date 1/2/11	Valid period 2 days	12.00												
				14.00												
Signature R Dickinson		Dispensed 1/2/11		18.00												
				22.00												
Additional comments																

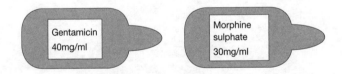

Gentamicin 40mg/ml

Morphine sulphate 30mg/ml

11. What dose of gentamicin does Davy require?

12. How many ampoules of gentamicin would you need to administer for Davy's 9am dose?

13. How many ampoules of morphine sulphate would you administer for Davy's 12pm dose?

14. Your colleague has prepared the medication for a patient and has prepared 4 tablets of digoxin 62.5mcg. The patient's prescription is for 500mcg. Is your colleague correct?

15. You need to prepare an injection of 6mg adrenaline for a patient. The adrenaline available is adrenaline 1:1000 in 1ml ampoules. How many ampoules do you need?

16. You need to administer chloramphenicol 50mg/kg daily in three divided doses. Your patient weighs 30kg and the capsules available are 250mg. How many capsules would you need to administer for each dose?

17. Your patient has been prescribed 3mg/kg daily of spironolactone in three divided doses. The patient weighs 25kg. The tablets available are 25mg. How many tablets does your patient require for each dose?

18. Your patient calls you over to check the medication that a colleague has given to him. The patient has 6 tablets of 5mg prednisolone. His prescription is for 25mg prednisolone. Has he been given the correct number of tablets? If not, what is the correct number he should have been administered?

19. Your patient requires 500mg carbemazepine in two divided dosages to be administered rectally. The suppository strength available is 125mg per suppository. How many do you need to administer for each dose?

20. Your patient requires 3g amoxicillin. The capsules available contain 250mg amoxicillin. How many capsules do you need to administer?

(Answers: page 239)

● Assessment 2 – Calculating and understanding simple medicine dosages

(based on Chapter 1)

1. The strength of a 1ml adrenaline ampoule is adrenaline 1:100. How many milligrams of adrenaline does this ampoule contain?
2. Your patient has been prescribed benzylpenicillin 300mg/kg in four divided dosages. Your patient weighs 12kg. How many milligrams benzylpenicillin does your patient require each dose?
3. You need to administer 160mg sotalol to your patient. The tablets available are 80mg. How many tablets do you need to administer?
4. The prescription for hyoscine butylbromide is for 0.6mg. The vials available are 400mcg/ml. How many vials do you need to administer?
5. Your patient has been prescribed isosorbide dinitrate 240mg in four divided dosages. The tablets available are 30mg. How many tablets do you need to administer for each dose?
6. A colleague has prepared medication for a patient and has taken out 4 phenytoin tablets ready to administer. The prescription for the patient is for 300mg phenytoin and the tablets available are 100mg. Has the right dose been prepared?
7. A baby you are caring for has been prescribed 100mg/kg azlocillin. The baby weighs 4kg. What dose of azlocillin does the baby require?
8. Your patient requires 1mg/kg azathioprine. Your patient weighs 75kg and the available tablets are 25mg. How many tablets do you need to administer?
9. The doctor has prescribed 60mg/kg cefuroxine in three divided doses for a child who weighs 22kg. What dose does the child require for each administration?
10. Your patient requires 2g erythromycin. The tablets available are 500mg. How many tablets do you need to administer?

Use the following medicine chart and available drug strengths to calculate questions 11–14:

Sunnydene and Reynold NHS Trust

Name: Ola Adebeye   **Hospital Number:** 0157758

Weight: 15kg   **Height:** 95cm

REGULAR PRESCRIPTIONS

Year 2011		Date & Month 1st February		Date Time																		
Drug Cefpodoxime				07.00																			
				09.00																			
Dose 80mg	Route PO	Start date 1/2/11	Valid period 14 days	12.00																			
				14.00																			
Signature R Dickinson		Dispensed 1/2/11		18.00																			
				22.00																			
Additional comments																							
Drug Paracetamol				07.00																			
				09.00																			
Dose 120mg	Route PO	Start date 1/2/11	Valid period 2 days	12.00																			
				14.00																			
Signature R Dickinson		Dispensed 1/2/11		18.00																			
				22.00																			
Additional comments																							
Year 2011		Date & Month 1st February		Date Time																		
Drug Phenytoin				07.00																			
				09.00																			
Dose 30mg	Route IM	Start date 1/2/11	Valid period 14 days	12.00																			
				14.00																			
Signature R Dickinson		Dispensed 1/2/11		18.00																			
				22.00																			
Additional comments																							

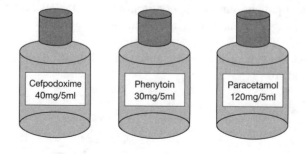

Cefpodoxime 40mg/5ml   Phenytoin 30mg/5ml   Paracetamol 120mg/5ml

11. You are due to give Ola her 9am medications. What medications is she due?

12. How many millilitres of the cefpodoxime dose available above does Ola require for her 9am dose?

13. How many millilitres of phenytoin suspension do you need to administer for Ola's 22:00hr dose?

14. How many millilitres of paracetamol will Ola need for her 12pm dose?

15. A baby is prescribed cefaclor 40mg/kg daily in four divided doses for a severe infection. The baby weighs 5kg. How many milligrams does the baby require for each dose?

16. You are asked to prepare 4mg adrenaline using adrenaline 1:1000 strength ampoules containing 1ml. How many millilitres do you need to make this dosage? How many ampoules is this?

17. Your colleague has prepared four tablets of amoxicillin 250mg for a patient. The prescription is for 1g. Has your colleague prepared the correct number of tablets for this dose?

18. You need to administer cefadroxil 25mg/kg to a child you are caring for in three divided dosages. How many milligrams do you need to administer for each dose if the child weighs 7.8kg?

19. Your patient is due to commence on phenytoin. The dose required is 4mg/kg daily in two divided dosages. Your patient weighs 37.5kg. The tablets available are 50mg and 25mg. How many of each tablet strength do you need to administer for each dose?

20. Your patient has been prescribed 3g metformin in three divided dosages. The tablets available are 500mg. How many tablets will your patient require for each dose?

(Answers: page 240)

● Assessment 3 – Medicines expressed as weight/ volume strengths

(based on Chapter 2)

1. You need to administer 62.5mg flucloxicillin orally to your patient. The suspension available contains 125mg/5ml. How many millilitres do you need to administer?

2. Your patient is in pain and requires oramorph. On his medicine chart he has been prescribed 20mg every 4 hours and is due a dose now. The oramorph suspension available is 10mg/5ml. How many millilitres do you need to administer?

3. Your patient has been prescribed morphine sulphate 15mg. The ampoules available are 20mg/2ml. How many millilitres do you need to administer?

4. The child you are caring for requires 50mg/kg amoxicillin daily in three divided doses. The weight for the child is 18kg. The suspension available contains 250mg/5ml. How many millilitres of this suspension do you need to administer for each dose?

5. Your patient has been prescribed gentamicin 2mg/kg IM. The patient weighs 78kg. The ampoules available contain 40mg/ml. How many millilitres do you need to administer?

6. You need to administer 25mg/kg co-amoxiclav intravenously to a baby who weighs 3kg. The co-amoxiclav vial contains 600mg. The displacement value for co-amoxiclav is 0.5ml and the final diluting volume required is 10ml. How many millilitres of water for injection do you need to reconstitute this drug with? How many millilitres do you need to administer?

7. You need to administer propranolol 80mg orally. The suspension available contains 40mg/5ml. How many millilitres do you need to administer?

8. Your patient has been prescribed amoxicillin 3g. The suspension available is 250mg/5ml. How many millilitres do you need to administer?

9. You need to administer 36mg/kg daily in two divided dosages to your patient. Your patient weighs 26kg. The suspension available contains 240mg/5ml. How many millilitres do you need to administer for each dose?

10. You need to administer diclofenac sodium 75mg IM to your patient. The ampoules contain 25mg/ml. How many millilitres do you need to administer?

Use the following medicine chart and medication strengths to answer questions 11–15:

Sunnydene and Reynold NHS Trust

Name: Sylvie Delort **Hospital Number:** 0056614

Weight: 18kg **Height:** 125cm

REGULAR PRESCRIPTIONS

Year 2011		Date & Month 1st February		Date Time													
Drug **Clarithromycin**				07.00													
				(09.00)													
Dose 187.5mg	Route PO	Start date 1/2/11	Valid period 14 days	12.00													
				14.00													
Signature R Dickinson		Dispensed 1/2/11		18.00													
				(22.00)													
Additional comments																	
Drug **Co-amoxiclav**				(07.00)													
				09.00													
Dose 25mg/kg	Route IV	Start date 1/2/11	Valid period 2 days	12.00													
				(14.00)													
Signature R Dickinson		Dispensed 1/2/11		18.00													
				(22.00)													
Additional comments																	
Year 2011		Date & Month 1st February		Date Time													
Drug **Paracetamol**				(07.00)													
				(09.00)													
Dose 240mg	Route PO	Start date 1/2/11	Valid period 14 days	12.00													
				14.00													
Signature R Dickinson		Dispensed 1/2/11		(18.00)													
				22.00													
Additional comments																	

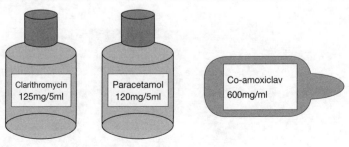

Clarithromycin
125mg/5ml

Paracetamol
120mg/5ml

Co-amoxiclav
600mg/ml

11. What medication is Sylvie due at 9am?
12. How many millilitres of clarithromycin do you need to administer?
13. How many millilitres of co-amoxiclav do you need to administer?
14. What syringe size would you choose to draw up this volume?
15. How many millilitres of paracetamol does Sylvie require?
16. Your patient requires 150mg oramorph. The suspension available is 100mg/5ml. How many millilitres do you need to administer?
17. A colleague has prepared an IM injection of morphine sulphate in a syringe for a patient (see below). The patient requires 15mg morphine sulphate and the strength of morphine used was 60mg/2ml. Has your colleague prepared the correct dose?

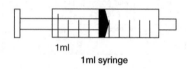

1ml
1ml syringe

18. Your patient requires phenytoin 150mg. The suspension available is 30mg/5ml. How many millilitres do you need to administer?
19. Your patient has been prescribed 2.4g benzylpenicillin IV. The ampoules available are 600mg. How many ampoules do you need to administer?
20. You need to administer 5mg adrenaline to your patient. The ampoules available are adrenaline 1:100 (1ml ampoules). How many millilitres do you need to administer?

(Answers: page 241)

● **Assessment 4 – Medicines expressed as weight/ volume strengths**

(based on Chapter 2)

1. Your patient requires 1g paracetamol. The suspension available contains 250mg/5ml. How many millilitres do you need to administer?
2. You need to administer 2mg/kg gentamicin IM to your patient. Your patient weighs 72kg. The ampoules available are 40mg/ml. How many millilitres do you need to administer?
3. Your patient has been prescribed 750mg amoxicillin orally. The suspension available is 125mg/5ml. How many millilitres do you need to administer?
4. You need to administer 6mg adrenaline IV. The ampoules available are adrenaline 1:100 (1ml). How many millilitres do you need to administer?
5. The baby you are caring for requires flucloxacillin 62.5mg IV. The ampoules contain 250mg in powder form. The displacement volume for a 250mg ampoule is 0.2ml and the diluting volume required is 5ml. How many millilitres do you need to reconstitute the flucloxacillin with? How many millilitres would you administer?
6. Your patient has been prescribed 250mcg/kg prochlorperazine orally. Your patient weighs 12kg. The suspension available is 5mg/5ml. How many millilitres do you need to administer?
7. Your patient has been prescribed metoclopramide 2mg IV. The ampoule strength available is 5mg/ml. How many millilitres do you need to administer?
8. You need to administer 150mg phenytoin. The suspension available is 30mg/5ml. How many millilitres do you need to administer?
9. Your colleague has prepared 20ml erythromycin suspension of strength 125mg/5ml for a patient. The patient has been prescribed 1g erythromycin. Is this the correct volume to administer?
10. Your patient requires 8mg ondansetron. The suspension available is 4mg/5ml. How many millilitres do you need to administer?

Use the following medication chart and medication strengths to answer questions 11–14:

Sunnydene and Reynold NHS Trust

Name: Jemaine Bent   **Hospital Number:** 001143254

Weight: 15.6kg   **Height:** 125cm

REGULAR PRESCRIPTIONS

Year 2011		Date & Month 1st February		Date Time												
Drug Metoclopramide				07.00												
				09.00												
Dose 1mg	Route PO	Start date 1/2/11	Valid period 14 days	12.00												
				14.00												
Signature R Dickinson		Dispensed 1/2/11		18.00												
				22.00												
Additional comments																
Drug Sodium valporate				07.00												
				09.00												
Dose 20mg/kg	Route IV	Start date 1/2/11	Valid period 2 days	12.00												
				14.00												
Signature R Dickinson		Dispensed 1/2/11		18.00												
				22.00												
Additional comments																
Year 2011		Date & Month 1st February		Date Time												
Drug Morphine sulphate				07.00												
				09.00												
Dose 2.5mg	Route SC	Start date 1/2/11	Valid period 14 days	12.00												
				14.00												
Signature R Dickinson		Dispensed 1/2/11		18.00												
				22.00												
Additional comments																

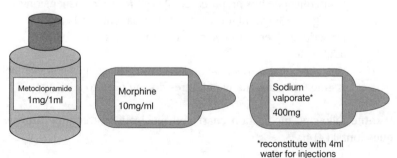

Metoclopramide 1mg/1ml

Morphine 10mg/ml

Sodium valporate* 400mg

*reconstitute with 4ml water for injections

11. What medications is Jemaine due at 7am?
12. How many millilitres of morphine do you need to draw up to administer for Jemaine?
13. How many millilitres of sodium valporate do you need to administer?
14. How many millilitres of metoclopramide do you need to administer for Jemaine's 14:00hr dose?
15. Your patient requires 200mcg/kg morphine SC. Your patient weighs 9.8kg, the ampoules available are 1mg/1ml. How many millilitres do you need to administer?
16. You need to administer 0.6mg hyoscine butylbromide to your patient. The ampoules available are 400mcg/ml. How many millilitres do you need to administer?
17. A patient asks you to check the amount of cefuroxime suspension they have been administered. The volume prepared is 10ml. The patient has been prescribed 250mg and the suspension strength available is 125mg/5ml. Has the patient been administered the correct amount?
18. You need to administer benzylpenicllin 50mg/kg daily in four divided doses to your patient. Your patient weights 1.2kg. The ampoules available are 600mg. The displacement volume is 0.4ml and the total diluting volume required is 5ml. How many millilitres would you reconstitute the benzylpenicillin with? How many millilitres would you administer?
19. Your patient has been prescribed 8500 units of clexane. The prefilled syringe contains 10 000 units/1ml. How many millilitres do you need to administer?
20. Your patient requires 5mg/kg of vancomycin IV. Your patient weighs 14.8kg. The ampoules available contain125mg (dilute with 10ml water for injection). How many millilitres do you need to administer?

(Answers: page 241)

● Assessment 5 – Calculations involving continuous infusions

(based on Chapter 3)

1. Your patient has been prescribed 1L 0.9% sodium chloride to be infused over 8 hours. You have a volumetric infusion device available which requires the rate to be programmed as ml/hr. What rate should you set this infusion for?

2. A 500ml 5% glucose infusion has been prescribed to be infused over 6 hours. Using a volumetric infusion device that requires the rate to be programmed as ml/hr, what rate would you set this infusion for?

Use the following IV medicine chart to calculate the following infusion rates using a manual giving set with a drop factor of 20 drops/ml (questions 3–7):

Date prescribed	Solution	Volume	Duration of infusion	Date to be given	Prescriber's signature
1/2/2011	5% glucose	1000ml	12 hours	1/2/2011	R Dickenson
1/2/2011	0.9% sodium chloride	1000ml	8 hours	2/2/2011	R Dickenson
1/2/2011	4% glucose, 0.18% sodium chloride (dextrose saline)	500ml	6 hours	2/2/2011	O A Adebeye

3. How many drops per minute would you set the 5% glucose infusion for?

4. Calculate the drops per minute required for the 0.9% sodium chloride infusion.

5. Calculate the drops per minute that you would set the infusion for the dextrose saline.

6. How many grams of glucose are contained in the dextrose saline infusion?

7. How many grams of sodium chloride are contained in the 0.9% sodium chloride infusion?

8. Your patient has been prescribed heparin 30 000 units/50ml over 24 hours. The stock ampoules of heparin available are 50 000 units/ml. How many millilitres of this ampoule would you need for the infusion? If you set this infusion rate as 4ml/hr, how many units of heparin would your patient be receiving every hour?

9. You set up an infusion of dopamine containing 80mg/50ml and set the rate as 5ml/hr. How many milligrams of the drug is the patient receiving per hour?

10. Your patient needs to be administered 0.2mcg/kg/min of a drug. Your patient's weight is 55kg. The infusion used in your clinical area is 12mg/50ml. Calculate the rate per hour you would set this infusion up for (ml/hr).

11. You need to add 4mmol potassium to an infusion of 0.9% sodium chloride. The ampoules of potassium available are 20mmol/10ml. How many millilitres of this ampoule do you need to add to the infusion bag?

12. Your patient has been prescribed 50 units actrapid/50ml and requires 2 units per hour administered initially. What rate would you set this infusion for (ml/hr)?

13. You need to administer 1mcg/kg/min of a drug. The infusion available is 800mg/500ml and your patient weights 67kg. How many millilitres per hour would you set this infusion for?

14. Your patient has been written up for the following prescription:

Prescription		Stock ampoules available
morphine sulphate 60mg	administered over	morphine sulphate 60mg/2ml
midazolam 10mg	24 hours via a	midazolam 10mg/2ml
levomepromazine 25mg	syringe driver	levomepromazine 25mg/1ml

Calculate the number of millilitres of the available stock ampoules for each drug. Using a 1-hour syringe driver, what rate (mm/hr) would you set this driver for?

15. Your patient has been prescribed aminophylline 500mcg/kg/hour. The standard infusion for your clinical area is 500mg/500ml. Your patient weighs 57kg. What rate per hour would you set the infusion for (ml/hr)?

16. Your patient has been prescribed heparin 100 units/kg/hour. Your patient weighs 50kg. How many units of heparin are required for a continuous infusion over 24 hours? The ampoules available are 50 000 units/ml. How many millilitres do you need to administer?

17. Your patient requires 5mcg/kg/min dopamine. The standard infusion for your clinical area is 80mg/50ml. Your patient weighs 28kg. What rate per hour do you need to set this infusion for (ml/hr)?

18. Your patient has been written up for the following prescription:

Prescription		Stock ampoules available
morphine sulphate 240mg hyoscine butylbromide 0.6mg midazolam 25mg	} administered over 24 hours via a syringe driver	morphine sulphate 60mg/1ml hyoscine butylbromide 400mcg/1ml midazolam 10mg/2ml

Calculate the number of millilitres of the available stock ampoules for each drug. What syringe size do you need to use for this infusion? Using a 1-hour syringe driver, what rate (mm/hr) would you set this driver for?

19. You need to administer amoxicillin 50mg/kg to a patient in four divided dosages. The ampoules available are 250mg in powder form. The displacement value for amoxicillin is 0.2ml and the diluting volume required is 10ml. Your patient weighs 1.2kg. How many millilitres of dilutent would you use and how many millilitres of the ampoule would you administer?

20. Your patient has been prescribed aminophylline 500mcg/kg/hour. The standard infusion for your clinical area is 500mg/500ml. Your patient weighs 35kg. What rate per hour would you set the infusion for (ml/hr)?

(Answers: page 242)

● **Assessment 6 – Calculations involving continuous infusions**

(based on Chapter 3)

1. Your patient has been prescribed 1000ml 5% glucose to be infused over 8 hours. What rate per hour (ml/hr) would you set this infusion for using a volumetric infusion device?

2. You need to set up an infusion for 0.9% sodium chloride 500ml to run over 6 hours. Using a volumetric infusion device, what rate per hour (ml/hr) would you programme the device for?

3. Your patient has been prescribed 100ml 0.9% sodium chloride with 2mmol potassium to be infused over 4 hours. The potassium ampoules available are 20mmol/10ml. How many millilitres of the potassium ampoule do you need to administer? What rate (ml/hr) would you set this infusion for using a volumetric infusion device?

Using the IV medicine chart below and a giving set that has 15 drops/ml, answer questions 4–8:

Date prescribed	Solution	Volume	Duration of infusion	Date to be given	Prescriber's signature
1/2/2011	gelofusine	500ml	2 hours	1/2/2011	R Dickenson
1/2/2011	1 unit blood	500ml	4 hours	2/2/2011	R Dickenson
1/2/2011	5% glucose	500ml	6 hours	2/2/2011	O A Adebeye

4. How many drops per minute would you set the gelofusine infusions for?

5. How many drops per minute would you set the unit of blood for?

6. How many grams of glucose are contained in the glucose infusion?

7. Calculate the drops per minute required for the glucose infusion?

8. The gelofusine infusion contains 4% gelatine. How many grams of gelofusine are contained in this 500ml infusion?

9. A patient has an infusion of insulin running that contains 50 units actrapid in 50ml. The infusion is currently running at 3ml/hr. How many units of insulin is this patient receiving currently?

10. An infusion of heparin contains 25 000 units/50ml. The infusion is required over 24 hours. What rate would you set the infusion for and how many units of heparin would the patient be receiving per hour? (n.b. 2ml volume used for priming the infusion line)

11. An aminophyline infusion is always set up containing 500mg/500ml. Your patient has been prescribed 500mcg/kg/hour. Your patient weighs 57.8kg. What rate would you set the infusion for (ml/hr)?

12. A colleague has prepared an infusion of heparin containing 50 000 units/50ml and tells you that they are going to set the rate for 4ml/hr. The prescription for the patient was for 4000 units of heparin per hour. Has your colleague prepared the correct dose?

13. Your patient has been written up for the following prescription:

Prescription		Stock ampoules available
morphine sulphate 120mg hyoscine butylbromide 0.6mg clonazepam 1mg	administered over 24 hours via a syringe driver	morphine sulphate 60mg/1ml hyoscine butylbromide 400mcg/1ml clonazepam 1mg/1ml

Calculate the number of millilitres of the available stock ampoules for each drug. Using a 1-hour syringe driver, what rate (mm/hr) would you set this driver for?

14. Your patient requires 5mcg/kg/min dopamine. The standard infusion for your clinical area is 80mg/50ml. Your patient weighs 35.8kg. What rate (ml) per hour do you need to set this infusion for?

15. Your patient needs to be administered 0.4mcg/kg/min of a drug. Your patient's weight is 35.5kg. The infusion used in your area is 12mg/50ml. Calculate the rate per hour (ml/hr) you would set this infusion up for.

16. Your colleague wants to set the rate for an aminophylline infusion (500mg/500ml) as 3.4ml/hr. The patient has been prescribed 500mcg/kg/hour and weighs 77.8kg. Is your colleague correct?

17. You need to administer amoxicillin 50mg/kg to a patient in four divided dosages. The ampoules available are 250mg in powder form. The displacement value for amoxicillin is 0.2ml and the diluting volume required is 10ml. Your patient weighs 0.8kg. What volume do you need to dilute the amoxicillin with and how many millilitres of the ampoule would you administer?

18. Your patient has been written up for the following prescription:

Prescription		Stock ampoules available
morphine sulphate 240mg haloperidol 1.5mg hyoscine butylbromide 0.2mg	administered over 24 hours via a syringe driver	morphine sulphate 60mg/1ml haloperidol 5mg/1ml hyoscine butylbromide 400mcg/1ml

Calculate the number of millilitres of the available stock ampoules for each drug. Using a 1-hour syringe driver, what rate (mm/hr) would you set this driver for?

19. Your patient requires 2mcg/kg/min dopamine. The standard infusion for your clinical area is 80mg/50ml. Your patient weighs 16.8kg. What rate per hour do you need to set this infusion for (ml/hr)?

20. Your patient requires an insulin infusion over 24 hours. This is set at 50 units of actrapid/50ml. Your patient's current blood glucose reading is 15.2mmol/L. Using the sliding scale below, what rate (ml/hr) would you set the infusion for?

Blood glucose (mmol/L)	Insulin infusion rate (mls/hr)
0.4	0.5
4.1–7	1
7.1–11	2
11.1–15	3
15.1–20	4
< 20	6 and call doctors to review scale

(Answers: page 242)

● **Assessment 7 – Calculations specific to acute nursing**

1. You need to administer 1.2g benzylpenicillin IV to your patient. The ampoules available are 600mg. How many ampoules do you need to administer?

2. Your patient has been prescribed 0.6mg hyoscine butylbromide. The ampoules available are 400mcg/1ml. How many millilitres do you need to administer?

3. You need to administer 0.125mg digoxin orally to your patient. The tables available are 62.5mcg. How many tablets do you need to administer?

4. You need to administer amoxicillin 500mg orally to your patient. The suspension available is 125mg/5ml. What volume of this suspension do you need to administer?

Use the following IV medication chart to calculate the questions 5–8 using a volumetric infusion device (ml/hr):

Date prescribed	Solution	Volume	Duration of infusion	Date to be given	Prescriber's signature
1/2/2011	5% glucose	1000ml	8 hours	1/2/2011	R Dickenson
1/2/2011	0.9% sodium chloride	1000ml	10 hours	2/2/2011	R Dickenson
1/2/2011	dextrose saline	1000ml	12 hours	2/2/2011	O A Adebeye

5. Calculate the rate (ml/hr) of the glucose infusion.
6. Calculate the rate (ml/hr) of the sodium chloride infusion.
7. Calculate the rate (ml/hr) of the dextrose saline infusion.
8. Dextrose saline contains 4% glucose and 0.18% sodium chloride. Calculate the number of grams of glucose and sodium chloride contained in the 1000ml infusion.
9. A patient has been prescribed aminophylline 500mcg/kg/hour. The standard infusion in your ward is 500mg/500ml. Your patient weighs 56.7kg. What rate per hour do you need to set the infusion for (ml/hr)?
10. Your patient has been prescribed 7.5mg/kg clarithromycin. Your patient weighs 5.2kg. The suspension contains 125mg/5ml. How many millilitres do you need to administer?
11. Your patient has been prescribed vancomycin IV 10mg/kg. Your patient weighs 12.5kg. What dose does your patient need? The vancomycin vial contains 250mg. You need to dilute the

ampoule with 10ml water for injection and the displacement value is 0.4ml. How many millilitres of water for injection do you need to add and how many millilitres do you need to administer?

Use the following medicine chart and medication strengths below to calculate questions 12–15:

Sunnydene and Reynold NHS Trust

Name: Lotte Clancy   **Hospital Number:** 03145274

Weight: 56.6kg   **Height:** 165cm

REGULAR PRESCRIPTIONS

Year 2011		Date & Month 1st February		Date Time													
Drug Phenytoin				07.00													
				09.00													
Dose 30mg	Route PEG	Start date 1/2/11	Valid period 14 days	12.00													
				14.00													
Signature R Dickinson		Dispensed 1/2/11		18.00													
				(22.00)													
Additional comments																	
Drug Flucloxacilin				(07.00)													
				09.00													
Dose 250mg	Route PEG	Start date 1/2/11	Valid period 2 days	12.00													
				(14.00)													
Signature R Dickinson		Dispensed 1/2/11		(18.00)													
				(22.00)													
Additional comments																	
Year 2011		Date & Month 1st February		Date Time													
Drug Morphine sulphate				(07.00)													
				09.00													
Dose 20mg	Route IM	Start date 1/2/11	Valid period 14 days	(12.00)													
				14.00													
Signature R Dickinson		Dispensed 1/2/11		(18.00)													
				(22.00)													
Additional comments																	

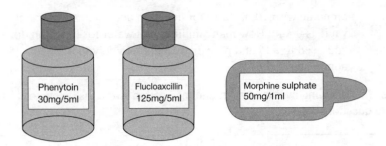

12. How many millilitres of phenytoin do you need to administer for Lotte's 10pm dose?

13. How many millilitres of the morphine ampoule does Lotte require?

14. How many millilitres of flucloxacillin does Lotte require?

15. What drugs is Lotte due at 7am?

16. You need to administer 8mg adrenaline IV. The ampoules available are adrenaline 1:100 (1ml). How many millilitres do you need to administer?

17. Your patient has been prescribed amoxicillin 375mg in three divided doses. How many milligrams does your patient require for each dose?

18. You patient has been prescribed 0.9% sodium chloride 1000ml to be infused over 10 hours manually. The giving set has a drop factor of 20 drops/ml. How many drips per minute do you need to set this infusion for?

19. Your patient requires 2mcg/kg/min dopamine. The standard infusion for your clinical area is 80mg/50ml. Your patient weighs 50.8kg. What rate per hour do you need to set this infusion for (ml/hr)?

20. Your colleague tells you that they are going to set an infusion of heparin 25 000 units/50ml at 2ml/hr. The patient has been prescribed 1000 units per hour. Is this the correct rate?

(Answers: page 243)

● Assessment 8 – Calculations specific to community nursing

1. You need to administer 0.125mg digoxin. The tablets available are 62.5mcg. How many tablets do you need to administer?

2. Your patient requires 500mg amoxicillin to be administered via a PEG. The elixir strength available is 125mg/5ml. How many millilitres (mls) would you administer?

Use the following information to calculate questions 3–5:

Your patient's pain is not being controlled. You discuss with the palliative care team who suggest that he takes a short-acting morphine, as required, and keeps a record of how much he has taken over 24 hours. The dose required to control his pain over 24 hours can then be used to calculate a slow-acting dose of morphine.

Your patient has been prescribed 50mg oramorph to be taken as required. The solution available is 100mg/5ml.

3. How many millilitres (mls) will your patient need to take to give a 50mg dose?

4. Your patient has taken 20ml of the oramorph which has 100mg/5ml strength in a 24-hour period. How many milligrams (mg) of oramorph has this patient taken in 24 hours?

5. You need to calculate the strength of MST Continus that your patient needs. MST Continus is a long-acting morphine tablet which works over 12 hours and is therefore taken twice daily. Using the total morphine dosage above, what strength would you recommend to be prescribed twice daily?

6. Your patient has been written up for the following prescription:

Prescription		Stock ampoules available
morphine sulphate 360mg midazolam 10mg hyoscine butylbromide 0.6mg	} administered over 24 hours via a syringe driver	morphine sulphate 60mg/ml midazolam 10mg/2ml hyoscine butylbromide 400mcg/1ml

Calculate the number of millilitres of the available stock ampoules for each drug. What syringe size would you use? Using a 1-hour syringe driver, what rate (mm/hr) would you set this driver for?

7. Your patient has been prescribed 2mg/kg of gentamicin IM. The patient's weight is 40kg. The ampoules available are 40mg/1ml. How many millilitres (mls) would you administer?

8. Your patient has been prescribed 80mg of a drug. The ampoules available are 200mg/2ml. How many millilitres (mls) would you administer from this ampoule?

9. A colleague has prepared 20ml phenytoin (30mg/5ml). The patient requires 150mg. Has your colleague prepared the correct volume?

10. You need to add 600mcg hyoscine to a patient's syringe driver. The ampoules available are 400mcg/ml? How many millilitres (mls) would you administer?

11. You need to administer 1g flucloxacillin. The tablets available are 500mg. How many do you need to administer?

12. Your patient has a syringe driver which contains 180mg of morphine sulphate over 24 hours. You need to administer one-sixth of the 24-hour dose to your patient subcutaneously (s/c) for breakthrough pain. What dose of morphine do you need to administer for breakthrough pain? The ampoules available are 50mg/ml. How many millilitres (mls) would you administer?

Your patient has been prescribed 200mcg salbutamol, 4 times daily. If the inhaler releases 100mcg per puff, use this information to answer questions 13–15:

13. How many puffs should your patient take to make up the required dose of 200mcg?

14. If your patient has 4 doses per day how many micrograms of salbutamol will they receive per day?

15. Express the total daily dosage of salbutamol in milligrams (mg).

16. Your patient requires 150mg phenytoin suspension. The suspension strength available is 30mg/5ml. How many millilitres do you need to administer?

17. A patient requires 30mg morphine sulphate SC for breakthrough pain. The ampoules available contain 50mg/ml. What volume do you need to administer?

18. Your patient has been written up for the following prescription:

Prescription		Stock ampoules available
morphine sulphate 60mg	administered over	morphine sulphate 60mg/ml
midazolam 10mg	24 hours via a	midazolam 10mg/2ml
metoclopramide 10mg	syringe driver	metoclopramide 5mg/ml

Calculate the number of millilitres of the available stock ampoules for each drug. Using a 1-hour syringe driver, what rate (mm/hr) would you set this driver for?

19. You need to administer 8000 units of clexane SC to your patient. Clexane is available in prefilled syringes 10 000 units/1ml. How many millilitres of this syringe do you need to administer?

20. You need to administer flucloxacillin 1g IV. The vials available are 500mg. How many vials do you need to administer?

(Answers: page 244)

● Assessment 9 – Calculations specific to paediatric nursing

1. You are caring for a child who requires 62.5mg amoxicillin to be administered orally. The suspension available contains 125mg/5ml. How many millilitres do you need to administer of this suspension?

2. A baby requires 100mg/kg benzylpenicillin daily in two divided dosages. The baby weighs 1.8kg. How many milligrams of benzylpenicillin does the baby require for each dose?

3. You need to administer 240mg benzylpenicillin IV. The vials contain 600mg and have a displacement volume of 0.4ml. How many millilitres of water for injection do you need to add to the vial if the total volume needs to be 5ml? How many millilitres do you need to administer?

4. You need to set up an infusion of 5% glucose 500ml over 12 hours for a patient using a manual giving set. The drop factor of the giving set is 15 drops/ml. How many drips per minute would you set this infusion for?

5. You need to administer 154mcg/kg papaveretum SC to a child. The child's weight is 12.kg. The ampoule available contains 7.7mg/ml. What volume of this ampoule do you need to administer?

6. You need to give 60mg paracetamol to a baby. The oral solution available contains 120mg/5ml. How many millilitres do you need to administer?

7. Your patient has been prescribed 240mcg morphine. The ampoules available are 1mg/ml. How many millilitres do you need to administer?

Use the following medicine chart and medication strengths to answer questions 8–11:

Sunnydene and Reynold NHS Trust

Name: Zainab Pickering   **Hospital Number:** 001164414

Weight: 8.6kg   **Height:** 55cm

REGULAR PRESCRIPTIONS

Year 2011	Date & Month 1st February	Date Time														
Drug Cefoxitin		07.00														
		09.00														

Dose 80mg/kg	Route IV	Start date 1/2/11	Valid period 14 days	12.00												
				14.00												
Signature R Dickinson		Dispensed 1/2/11		18.00												
				22.00												
Additional comments																
Drug Ampicillin				07.00												
				09.00												
Dose 250mg	Route IV	Start date 1/2/11	Valid period 2 days	12.00												
				14.00												
Signature R Dickinson		Dispensed 1/2/11		18.00												
				22.00												
Additional comments																
Year 2011		Date & Month 1st February		Date / Time												
Drug Paracetamol				07.00												
				09.00												
Dose 125mg	Route PR	Start date 1/2/11	Valid period 14 days	12.00												
				14.00												
Signature R Dickinson		Dispensed 1/2/11		18.00												
				22.00												
Additional comments																

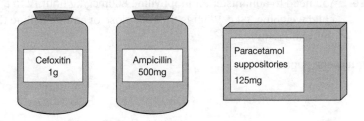

8. How many milligrams of cefoxitin does Zainab require each dose?
9. Using the vial strength above and a final diluting volume of 10ml, calculate how many millilitres of cefoxitin you need to administer.
10. How many millilitres of the ampicillin vial do you need to administer if the diluting volume is 10ml?
11. How many suppositories does Zainab require for each dose?
12. A 9-month-old baby you are caring for has been prescribed cefuroxime IV 200mg/kg in four divided dosages. The baby weighs 4.9kg. The vials available contain 250mg. The displacement volume is 0.2ml and the total diluting volume is 2ml. Calculate how many millilitres of this reconstituted vial you need to administer for each dose.

13. A child weighing 16.8kg requires 4mg/kg ranitidine orally. The suspension contains 75mg/5ml. How much do you need to administer?

14. A child requires an IV infusion of 0.9% sodium chloride 500ml to be infused over 10 hours. Calculate the rate to set a volumetric infusion device (ml/hr).

15. You need to add 12mmols potassium to an infusion. The potassium ampoules available contain 20mmol/10ml. How much of this ampoule do you need?

16. A child requires a dopamine infusion and has been prescribed 30mg/kg continuously over 24 hours. The child weighs 1.9kg. Calculate the dose of dopamine required for the 24 hours.

17. A baby has been prescribed morphine SC 150mcg/kg. The baby weighs 1.2kg. The ampoules available contain 1mg/ml. How much of this ampoule would you administer?

18. A child requires 0.8g cabemazepine in four divided dosages. The suspension contains 100mg/5ml. How much do you need to give each dose?

19. A colleague has prepared a syringe containing 4.8ml phenytoin (30mg/5ml). The child weighs 10.2kg and the prescription is for 5mg/kg in two divided dosages. Is your colleague correct?

20. You need to administer aminophylline 800mcg/kg/hour IV to a child weighing 38kg. What is the total dose of aminophylline that this child requires?

(Answers: page 244)

● **Assessment 10 – Calculations for adult nursing**

1. Your patient has been prescribed 1.8g benzylpenicillin. The vials available contain 600mg. How many vials do you require?

2. You need to administer 300mg phenytoin to a patient. The tablets available contain 100mg. How many tablets do you need to administer?

3. A colleague has prepared 1.5ml morphine sulphate (60mg/2ml) to administer to a patient. The patient has been prescribed 45mg morphine. Is you colleague correct?

Use the IV medicine chart to answer the following infusion questions (4–6) using a volumetric electronic device (ml/hr):

Date prescribed	Solution	Volume	Duration of infusion	Date to be given	Prescriber's signature
1/2/2011	gelofusine	500ml	1 hour	1/2/2011	R Dickenson
1/2/2011	5% glucose	500ml	4 hours	2/2/2011	R Dickenson
1/2/2011	dextrose saline	1000ml	4 hours	2/2/2011	O A Adebeye

4. What rate (ml/hr) would you set the gelofusine infusion for?

5. What rate (ml/hr) would you set the 5% glucose infusion for?

6. How many grams of glucose and sodium chloride are contained in the dextroxe saline infusion (4% glucose and 0.18% dextrose saline)?

7. You have been asked to prepare 0.5mg adrenaline for a patient using adrenaline 1:1000 strength (1ml). How many millilitres do you need to prepare?

8. Your patient has been prescribed aminophylline 500mcg/kg/hr. Your patient weighs 46.8kg. The aminophylline infusion in your clinical areas is always 500mg/500ml. What rate (ml/hr) do you need to set this infusion for?

9. You need to prepare a continuous infusion of heparin 75 000 units over 24 hours. The heparin ampoules available as stock are 100 000 units. How many millilitres of this ampoule do you need? What rate (ml/hr) would you set this infusion for (n.b. always 50ml)?

10. Your patient is on an insulin sliding scale and has an IV infusion of insulin containing 50 units actrapid/50ml. Your patient's blood glucose level is 9.7mmols/L. Using the sliding scale what rate does the infusion need to be running at?

Blood glucose (mmol/L)	Insulin infusion rate (mls/hr)
0.4	0.5
4.1–7	1
7.1–11	2
11.1–15	3
15.1–20	4
< 20	6 and call doctors to review scale

11. Your patient has been written up for the following prescription:

Prescription		Stock ampoules available
morphine 180mg	administered over 24 hours via a syringe driver	morphine sulphate 60mg/1ml
haloperidol 1.5mg		haloperidol 5mg/1ml
metoclopramide 10mg		metoclopramide 5mg/ml

Calculate the number of millilitres of the available stock ampoules for each drug. Using a 24-hour syringe driver, what rate (mm/hr) would you set this driver for?

12. Your patient has been written up for a 1000ml 5% glucose infusion to be infused over 12 hours. The manual giving set available has a drop factor of 20 drops/ml. Calculate the drips per minute you need to set this infusion for.

Use the following medicine chart and medication strengths to answer the questions 13–15:

Sunnydene and Reynold NHS Trust

Name: Jonty Smith **Hospital Number:** 001164414

Weight: 86kg **Height:** 176cm

REGULAR PRESCRIPTIONS

Year 2011		Date & Month 1st February		Date Time										
Drug _Gentamicin_				07.00										
				09.00										
Dose 2mg/kg	Route IM	Start date 1/2/11	Valid period 14 days	12.00										
				14.00										
Signature R Dickinson		Dispensed 1/2/11		18.00										
				22.00										
Additional comments														

Drug Amoxicillin				07.00									
				09.00									
Dose 1g	Route IV	Start date 1/2/11	Valid period 2 days	12.00									
				14.00									
Signature R Dickinson		Dispensed 1/2/11		18.00									
				22.00									
Additional comments													
Year 2011		Date & Month 1st February		Date Time									
Drug Digoxin				07.00									
				09.00									
Dose 0.5mg	Route PO	Start date 1/2/11	Valid period 14 days	12.00									
				14.00									
Signature R Dickinson		Dispensed 1/2/11		18.00									
				22.00									
Additional comments													

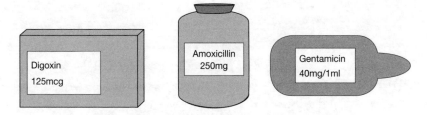

Digoxin 125mcg

Amoxicillin 250mg

Gentamicin 40mg/1ml

13. How many digoxin tablets should you administer?
14. How many vials of amoxicillin do you need to administer?
15. What volume of gentamicin do you need to administer?
16. You set up an infusion of dopamine containing 80mg/50ml and set the rate as 2.8ml/hr. How many milligrams of the drug is the patient receiving per hour?
17. Your patient has been written up for the following prescription:

Prescription		Stock ampoules available
morphine sulphate 120mg	administered over 24 hours via a syringe driver	morphine sulphate 60mg/1ml
midazolam 10mg		midazolam 10mg/ml
hyoscine butylbromide 0.6mg		hyoscine butylbromide 400mcg/ml

Calculate the number of millilitres of the available stock ampoules for each drug. Using a 24-hour syringe driver, what rate (mm/hr) would you set this driver for?

18. You need to administer cefuroxime 1.5g as a single dose. The vials available are 750mg. Assuming a diluting volume of 10ml for each 750 vial, how many millilitres would you administer?

19. Your patient requires 2mcg/kg/min dopamine. The standard infusion for your clinical area is 80mg/50ml. Your patient weighs 67.8kg. What rate per hour do you need to set this infusion for?

20. A colleague has prepared 20ml of carbemazepine. The patient has been prescribed 1.2g in four divided dosages. The suspension available is 100mg/5ml. Has your colleague prepared the correct dose?

(Answers: page 245)

Answers

No peeking until you're 100% sure of your solution!

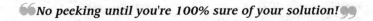

CHAPTER 1

EXERCISE 1

1. **Formula method**

$$\frac{\text{what you want}}{\text{what you have}} = \text{number of tablets}$$

$$\frac{1000 \text{ milligrams}}{250 \text{ milligrams}} = 4 \text{ tablets}$$

Repeated addition

250 milligrams	1 tablet
500 milligrams	2 tablets
750 milligrams	3 tablets
1000 milligrams	4 tablets

Or

250 milligrams	1 tablet
500 milligrams	2 tablets
1000 milligrams	4 tablets
	(doubling 500)

2. **Formula method**

$$\frac{\text{what you want}}{\text{what you have}} = \text{number of tablets}$$

$$\frac{250 \text{ micrograms}}{62.5 \text{ micrograms}} = 4 \text{ tablets}$$

Repeated addition

62.5 micrograms	1 tablet
125 micrograms	2 tablets
187.5 micrograms	3 tablets
250 micrograms	4 tablets

Or

62.5 micrograms	1 tablet
125 micrograms	2 tablets
250 micrograms	4 tablets

EXERCISE 2

Grams to milligrams

1. You know that 1 gram = 1000 milligrams. You need one thousand milligrams for every 1 gram. So you need to multiply the gram weight by one thousand to work out the equivalent milligram weight:

   0.6 grams x 1000 milligrams = 600
   Alternatively you could write down:
   1 gram = 1000 milligrams
   0.6 grams = ?
   And 'see' that the answer would be 600 milligrams.
   Finally, you might consider the example previously of 500 milligram tablets of paracetmol being 0.5g and work out that this is similar to 0.6, so would be 600 milligrams.

2. 1200 milligrams

3. 250 milligrams

Milligrams to grams

1. You know that 1000 milligrams = 1 gram. You need a thousand times less grams than milligrams. So you need to divide the milligram weight by one thousand to work out the equivalent gram weight:

   1800 milligrams ÷ 1000 = 1.8 grams
   Alternatively you could write down:
   1000 milligrams = 1 gram
   1800 milligrams = ?
   And see that the answer would be 1.8 grams.

Finally, you could use a drug dosage that you are familiar with. You may recognise that 1.8 grams and 1800 milligrams are common benzlypenicillin dosages and 'know' the conversion or you may be aware that 1000 milligrams paracetamol is 1 gram so 1800 milligrams must be 1.8 grams.

2. 0.8 grams

3. 2 grams

Milligrams to micrograms

1. You know that 1 milligram = 1000 micrograms. You need one thousand micrograms to equal the weight of 1 milligram. So you need one thousand times more micrograms to make the equivalent milligram weight. You therefore need to multiply the milligram weight by one thousand to work out the equivalent microgram weight:

   0.3 milligrams x 1000 = 300 micrograms

   Alternatively you could write down:
   1 milligram = 1000 micrograms
   0.3 milligrams = ?
   And see that the answer would be 300 micrograms.

   Finally, you could use a drug dosage that you know, such as hyoscine, and 'know' that 600 micrograms of hyoscine is 0.6 milligrams so 0.3 milligrams would be 300 micrograms.

2. 125 micrograms

3. 10 micrograms

Micrograms to milligrams

1. You know that 1000 micrograms = 1 milligram. You need a thousand times less milligrams than micrograms. So you need to divide the microgram weight by one thousand to work out the equivalent microgram weight:

100 micrograms ÷ 1000 = 0.1 milligrams

Alternatively you could write down:
1000 micrograms = 1 milligram
100 micrograms = ?

And see that the answer would be 0.1 milligrams.

2. 0.5 milligrams

3. 2.5 milligrams

EXERCISE 3

1. *Your patient has been prescribed 0.25 milligrams digoxin. The tablets available each contain 62.5 micrograms. How many tablets would you administer?*

   (a) *Think about what you are actually trying to work out, for example how many tablets to administer or how much of an ampoule to administer:*

   How many 62.5 microgram tablets need to be administered to give the prescribed dose of 0.25 milligrams?

   (b) *Check the units of measurement in prescribed dosage and available drug dosage are the same:*

   The prescribed dose is in milligrams and the available tablets are in micrograms so a conversion is required.

   (c) *If the units of measurement are different then convert the prescribed dosage units into the available drug units:*

   How many micrograms are there in 0.25 milligrams? Micrograms are smaller than milligrams so more of these are needed to make the required weight of 0.25 milligrams. One milligram is the same weight as 1000 micrograms.

I therefore need to multiply 0.25 milligrams by one thousand.

0.25 milligrams x 1000 = 250 micrograms

Or

1 milligram = 1000 micrograms

0.25 milligrams = 250 micrograms

(d) *Go back to the question and recheck what you are trying to work out using the new measurements:*

You need to give 250 micrograms. You have tablets available that each contains 62.5 micrograms. How many of these tablets will make up the required dosage of 250 micrograms?

(e) *Work out how many tablets or ampoules to administer using formula method or repeated addition:*

How many 62.5 micrograms tablets will give me 250 micrograms?

Formula method

$$\frac{\text{what I want to administer}}{\text{what I have available}}$$

$$\frac{250 \text{ micrograms}}{62.5 \text{ micrograms}} = 4 \text{ tablets}$$

Repeated addition

62.5 micrograms	1 tablet
125 micrograms	2 tablets
250 micrograms	4 tablets (125 multiplied by 2)

(f) *Check that your answer makes sense in relation to the question and clinical practice, for example is it usual in practice to give this number of tablets? Is this the usual number of tablets to give for this drug? If you gave this number of tablets what dosage would you be giving (add up the dosage for*

each tablet and check it is the same as the prescribed dosage):

Do I usually give 4 tablets in practice? *Yes, not usually, but sometimes.*

Is this the usual amount of digoxin administered? *Yes.*

If I were giving 4 tablets, each with a dosage of 62.5 micrograms, then 2 would be 125 micrograms and 4 would be 250 micrograms. *So yes, this is the right dosage.*

2. 2 ampoules

3. 4 tablets

4. 5 millilitres

5. Half of the ampoule

EXERCISE 4

1. 1:1000 adrenaline means that 1g adrenaline is in 1000ml. We need to convert the adrenaline dosage to milligrams and then calculate how many milligrams in 0.5ml:

1g in 1000ml	
1000mg in 1000ml	convert grams to milligrams
1mg in 1ml	divide by 1000
0.5mg in 0.5ml	halve

   The answer is 0.5mg.

2. 1:100 adrenaline means that 1g adrenaline is in 100ml. We need to convert the adrenaline dose to milligrams and then calculate how many milligrams are in 2ml:

1g in 100ml	
1000mg in 100ml	convert grams to milligrams
10mg in 1ml	divide by 100
20mg in 2ml	double

   The answer is 20mg.

3. 1:10 000 adrenaline means that 1g adrenaline is in 10 000ml. We need to

work out how many micrograms are in 1ml:

1g in 10 000ml

1000mg in 10 000ml	convert to milligrams
1mg in 10ml	divide both sides by 1000
1000mcg in 10ml	convert milligrams to micrograms
100mcg in 1ml	divide both sides by 10
200mcg in 2ml	double

You would need to administer 2ml.

EXERCISE 5

1. *Your patient has been prescribed 50mg/kg of amoxicillin. Your patient weighs 10kg. The amoxicillin ampoules available contain 250mg. How many of these ampoules do you need to administer to your patient in order to give the prescribed dosage?*

   (a) *Make sure you understand the question and what exactly you are trying to work out, for example dosage for the individual patient and then how much of the available drug to give in order to administer this dosage:*

   The dosage has been prescribed as the amount to administer for every kilogram weight of the patient. I need to work out what dosage my patient requires of amoxicillin using their weight and then, once I know this, I can work out what volume of the medicine contains this dosage.

   (b) *Calculate the individual dose for the patient by multiplying their weight in kilograms by the dosage per kilogram:*

   50mg x 10kg = 500mg

   (c) *Go back to the question and check that you are still clear about your understanding, for example I know the actual dosage, I now need to calculate how much of the available drug to administer:*

   My patient needs to be administered a dose of 500mg amoxicillin. The available ampoules contain 250mg so I need to work out how many would contain 500mg.

   (d) *Check that the prescribed dosage has the same unit of measurements as the available drug dosage:*

   Yes both dosages are in milligrams.

   (e) *If the units of measurement are different then convert the prescribed dosage so it is expressed in the same unit of measurement as the available drug:*

   Both units of measurement are the same.

   (f) *Go back to the question and check that you are still clear about your understanding, for example I need to administer this dosage, I have this dosage available and they are both now in the same unit of measurement. I now need to work out how much of this drug would give the prescribed dosage:*

   I still need to work out how many ampoules would contain the 500mg dosage.

   (g) *Work out how much of the available drug to administer by using repeated addition or dividing the prescribed dosage by the available dosage:*

   I know that the ampoules contain 250mg in every 1ml.

Formula method

what I want to give

what I have available = number of ampoules

$$\frac{500mg}{250mg} = 2 \text{ ampoules}$$

Repeated addition

250mg   1 ampoule

500mg   2 ampoules

(i) *Check your answer makes sense in relation to the questions and the dosages being prescribed and available, and your knowledge of clinical practice, for example does it seem reasonable to administer this amount of a drug? Have I ever administered this amount before? Is this the usual amount of ampoules/tablets that I administer for this particular drug? Check your working out:*

Does my answer make sense? 2 ampoules seems a reasonable dose and I have administered this dose amount before. I will also double-check my dosage for the patient. They need 50mg for every kilogram weight and my patient weighs 10 kilograms so I need 10 lots of 50, which is 500mg. I will double-check the amount to administer again, so 2 lots of 250mg would be 500mg, which would be 2 ampoules, so yes, I am happy that 2 ampoules is the correct amount to administer.

2. The patient's dose is 2mg x 60kg, which gives a total dosage of 120mg. The amount to administer using the available 40mg/1ml ampoules would be 3 ampoules.

3. The patient's dose is 500mcg x 10kg, which gives a total dosage of 5000mcg. This is 5mg when expressed in milligrams. The amount to administer using the available 10mg/ml ampoule would be half of this ampoule, which is 0.5ml.

EXERCISE 6

1. 125mg

2. 1800mg divided by 3 gives 600mg three times a day.

3. Total daily dose is 1g. I need to divide this by the number of dosages required which is two. First, I need to convert 1g to milligrams to get 1000mg. I then need to divide 1000mg by 2 to get the answer of 500mg twice a day.

Assessment 1 (Chapter 1)

1. 2 tablets

2. 360mg

3. 4 tablets

4. 4 tablets

5. 152mg

6. 6 tablets

7. 2 vials

8. 2 tablets each dose

9. 3 tablets

10. 2 capsules

CHAPTER 2

EXERCISE 7

1. The whole ampoule contains 40mg, so if I administer the whole ampoule, I would have given 40mg

2. 5ml

3. 2ml

4. 1ml

5. 5ml

EXERCISE 8

1. Millish requires 5mg of metoclopramide IM (intramuscularly). The ampoules contain 5mg/ml so you would need to administer the whole 1ml ampoule.

2. Millish requires 20mg and the ampoules contain 20mg/1ml so you would need to administer the whole 1ml ampoule.

EXERCISE 9

1. 1ml

2. 2.5ml

3. 0.5ml

4. 2.5ml

5. *Worked through answer:*
   50mg in 5ml
   25mg in 2.5ml
   50mg + 25mg = 75mg
   Therefore 75mg would be 5ml + 2.5ml
   I would administer 7.5ml.

EXERCISE 10

1. 10ml

2. 2ml

3. 10ml

4. *Worked through answer:*

50mg in 5ml	available dose
100mg in 10ml	doubling volume and weight
200mg in 20ml	doubling volume and weight

   You would administer 20ml.

5. 4ml

EXERCISE 11

1. 1.5ml

2. 5ml

3. 2.5ml

4. 1.5ml

5. *Worked through answer:*

60mcg in 1ml	
120mcg in 2ml	doubling
30mcg in 0.5ml	halving

   120mcg + 30mcg = 2ml + 0.5ml = 2.5ml

   You would need to administer 2.5ml

EXERCISE 12

1. 0.6ml

2. 2ml

3. 0.6ml

4. *Worked through answer:*

100mg in 2ml	available dose
10mg in 0.2ml	dividing volume and weight by 10
60mg in 1.2ml	multiplying volume and weight by 6

5. 2ml

EXERCISE 13

1. 150mg is three-quarters of 200mg, so you need to administer three-quarters of 10ml, which is 7.5ml.

2. 2mg is a third of 6mg, so you need to administer one-third of 3ml, which is 1ml.

3. 20mcg is one-fifth of 100mcg, so you need to administer one-fifth of 5ml, which is 1ml.

4. 3mg is three-fifths of 5mg so you need to administer three-fifths of 2ml, which is 1.2ml (three-fifths of 1ml is

0.6, so three-fifths of 2ml would be two times this amount).

5. 80mg is four-fifths of 100mg so you need to administer four-fifths of 2ml, which would be 1.6ml (four-fifths of 1ml is 0.8, so four-fifths of 2ml would be two times this amount).

EXERCISE 14

1. 0.6ml (6 measurements on a 1ml syringe)

2. 0.4ml (4 measurements on a 2ml syringe)

3. 0.8ml (8 measurements on a 2ml syringe)

4. 1.2ml (12 measurements on a 2ml syringe)

5. *Worked through answer:*

   There are 20 measurements on a 2ml syringe. If the ampoule contains 25mg, then I could divide this by 20 to work out that each measurement on the syringe would contain 1.25mg and each two measurements would be 2.5mg. I could either count up in 2.5mg for each two measurements until I get to 15mg, for example 2.5mg, 5mg, 7.5mg, 10mg, 12.5mg and 15mg, which would be six lots of two measurements on the syringe, or I could think that four measurements would give me 5mg, so I need another four to make 10mg and another four to give 15mg, so twelve measurements in total. The total volume would be 1.2ml.

EXERCISE 15

1. Solution is incorrect. 5ml of the solution would give 125mg. I need to administer 250mg, which is more than 125mg so I need to give a greater volume than 5ml, not a smaller volume. The solution should be 10ml.

2. The solution is correct for the prescribed dosage **but** I have never administered 15 ampoules of hyoscine. I would need to check this prescription with pharmacy or the doctor who prescribed the dose. This prescription has been written in error and should read 0.6mg.

3. Solution is correct. Four lots of 0.25ml would give 1ml and four lots of 5mg would give 20mg.

4. Solution is incorrect. The ampoule contains 25 000 units/ml, and the amount required is 15 000, which is three-fifths of 25 000 so would be 0.6ml.

5. Solution is correct. Using the doubling method 30mg/5ml, so 60mg/10ml and 120mg/20ml. I am expecting my solution therefore to be more than 20ml. The dosage required is five times more than the available dosage so I need five times the volume, which would be 25ml. This volume is reasonable for a phenytoin suspension.

EXERCISE 16

1. 5

2. 20

3. 10

4. 0.5 or $\frac{1}{2}$

5. 4

6. $\frac{5}{4}$

7. $\frac{1}{4}$

8. $\frac{3}{5}$

9. $\frac{1}{5}$

10. $\frac{9}{2}$

11. 7.5

12. 0.6

13. 0.2

14. 11.25

15. 21.5

EXERCISE 17

1. 1.4ml

2. 0.15ml

3. 2ml

4. 1.2

5. *Worked through answer:*

   <u>what you want</u>   x   what it's in
   what you have available

   <u>600</u> x 5 = <u>60</u> x 5 (dividing top and
   250   25   bottom by 10)
   <u>60</u> x 1 (dividing 5 and 25 by 5)
   5
   <u>60</u> x 1 = <u>60</u> = 12 (60 divided by 5)
   5   5

   Solution: I would administer 12 ml.

EXERCISE 18

1. Formula method would be useful. Could also use doubling to find out that 100mg/10ml and then reduce single unit to find out that 10mg/1ml therefore 42mg/4.2ml.

2. Using knowledge of patterns to see that 50mg is a quarter of 200mg so a quarter of the volume is required which is 0.5ml.

3. Using reducing down to single units to work out that 10mg/1ml and therefore 30mg/3ml. Answer would be 3ml.

4. Doubling would give 200mg/10ml and halving would give 50mg/2.5 ml. To administer 250ml, you would need therefore 10ml and 2.5ml so would need to administer 12.5ml.

5. You could use a 5ml syringe and work out that each 1ml measurement

would equal 20mg so you would need four lots of measurements which would be 4ml. Alternatively, you could use the reducing down to single units method to work out that 10mg/0.5ml by dividing by 10 and then multiply by 8 to work out 80mg/4ml or use the formula method.

EXERCISE 19

1. *Your patient has been prescribed 2mg/ kg gentamicin as an IM injection. Your patient weighs 72kg and the ampoules available are 40mg/ml. How many millilitres of this ampoule strength would you need to administer?*

   (a) *Make sure you understand the question and what exactly you are trying to work out, for example dosage for the individual patient and then how much of the available drug to give in order to administer this dosage:*

   You need to calculate the dose required for the patient according to body weight and then use this to calculate what volume from the ampoule contains this dose.

   (b) *Calculate the individual dose for the patient by multiplying their weight in kilograms by the dosage per kilogram:*

   72kg x 2 mg = 144mg

   (c) *Go back to the question and check that you are still clear about your understanding, for example I know the actual dosage, I now need to calculate how much of the available drug to administer:*

   I know that I need to administer 144mg. I now need to calculate how many millilitres of the ampoule strength 40mg/ml I need to administer to give this dose.

(d) *Check that the prescribed dosage has the same unit of measurements as the available drug dosage:*

The prescribed dose and available dose are both in milligrams.

(e) *If the units of measurement are different then convert the prescribed dosage so it is expressed in the same unit of measurement as the available drug:*

Not applicable.

(f) *Go back to the question and check that you are still clear about your understanding, for example I need to administer this dosage, I have this dosage available and they are both now in the same unit of measurement. I now need to work out what volume of this suspension, elixir or ampoule would give the prescribed dosage:*

No change to original understanding in answer to (c).

(g) *Examine the dosages in the question and decide which method would be best to solve the calculation. If you are unsure start with doubling and halving or use the formula method:*

I cannot see any pattern immediately between 144mg and 40mg so I will use the formula method.

(h) *Work out how much of the available drug to administer by using your chosen methods:*

$$\frac{144mg}{40mg} \times 1ml = \frac{72}{20} = \frac{36}{10} = \frac{18}{5} =$$

3 and $^{3}/_{5}$ which is same as 3.6ml

(i) *Check your answer makes sense in relation to the questions and the dosages being prescribed and available, and your knowledge of*

clinical practice, for example does it seem reasonable to administer this amount of a drug? Have I ever administered this amount before? Is this the usual volume that I administer for this particular drug?

I need to administer 144mg and each ampoule contains 40mg/ml. If I administered 3 ampoules that would be a dose of 40mg x 3 = 120mg. Half an ampoule would be 20mg/0.5ml. Administering 140mg would be 3.5ml so the answer of 3.6ml would be 3 ampoules and just over half of the fourth ampoule, which makes sense for 144mg.

(j) *If you are unsure, check through your work or use a different method. If you are still unsure you need to ask for help.*

Another method is the single unit method and doubling/halving:

40mg in 1ml
120mg in 3ml   multiplying by 3
20mg in 0.5ml   halving
2mg in 0.05   dividing by 10
4mg in 0.1   multiplying by 2
120mg + 20mg + 4mg = 3ml + 0.5ml + 1ml = 3.6ml

2. *You need to administer 5mg/kg phenytoin to your patient in two divided doses orally. The suspension available is 30mg/5ml. You patient's weight is 16.8kg. How many millilitres would you administer for each dose?*

Calculate dose for individual patient 16.8kg x 5mg = 84mg. This would be 42mg in two doses. You need to work out how many millilitres of 30mg/5ml strength contains 42mg. Using formula 42mg/30mg x 5ml = 7ml.

3. *The prescription for your patient is for 3g amoxicillin every 12 hours orally. You need to give the first dose of this*

drug to your patient. The suspension available is 250mg/5ml. How many millilitres do you need to administer?

First, convert the prescription dose to milligrams so you need to administer 3000mg amoxicillin. You then need to calculate how many millilitres of 250mg/5ml solution you would need in order to administer 3000mg. This would be 3000mg/250mg x 5ml or knowing that 4 lots of 250mg would make 1000mg so you need 4 lots of 5ml for 1000mg = 20ml. You can then multiply this by 3 to calculate 3000mg = 60ml.

4. *Your patient has been prescribed 1.5mg/kg frusemide orally. The paediatric liquid available is 1mg/1ml. How many millilitres would you need to administer to your patient who weighs 4kg?*

1.5mg x 4kg = 6mg dose for this patient. 1mg in 1ml, so 6mg in 6ml.

You would need to administer 6ml.

5. *You need to administer 0.25mg digoxin to your patient. The elixir available contains 50mcg/ml. How many millilitres do you need to administer?*

First, convert the prescribed dose to milligrams to make 250mcg (multiply 0.25 by 1000). You now need to calculate what volume of 50mcg/1ml would give 250mcg. This would be five lots of 50mcg so would be five lots of 1ml = 5ml.

EXERCISE 20

1. Solution strength would be 250mg/5ml.

2. Solution strength would be 500mg/10ml.

3. Solution strength would be 600mg/10ml.

EXERCISE 21

1. Administer all of the 10ml.

2. Administer 2ml.

3. Administer 2.5ml or half of the 5 ml syringe.

4. *Worked through answer:*

Firstly, you need the knowledge that you can only give 2ml or less as a subcutaneous injection so you need to ensure that the amount needing administration is less than this. The amount prescribed, 10mg, is half of the amount available, 20mg. Therefore you need to give half of any volume used to reconstitute the powder. You could reconstitute with 1ml and give 0.5ml, reconstitute with 2ml and give 1ml or reconstitute with 4ml and give 2ml.

5. Administer 1.6ml.

Assessment 2 (Chapter 2)

1. Jerome requires 30mg of frusemide IM. The ampoules contain 10mg/ml so you would need to administer 3 ampoules.

2. Jerome requires 15mg and the ampoules contain 30mg/2ml so you would need to administer half of the 1ml ampoule.

3. Akiko requires 250mg amoxicillin and the suspension contains 125mg/5ml. You would need to administer two lots of 125mg to give 250mg, which is 10ml.

4. Akiko requires 0.25g paracetamol and the available suspension strength is 250mg/5ml. You need to convert 0.25g into milligrams by multiplying by 1000 to get 250mg. You therefore need to administer 5ml.

5. *Worked through answer:*

First, you need to calculate the dose Jane requires by multiplying the dose per kg weight by Jane's weight which is on the top of the medicine chart and is 12.5kg. You need to work out 30mg x 12.5kg. You can either do this on the calculator, using long multiplication or by calculating 3 x 12 = 36, therefore 30mg x 12 = 360mg plus a half of 30mg = 15mg. Therefore 360mg + 15mg = 375mg.

You now know that Jane requires 375mg dose of cefuroxime. The vials of cefuroxime each contain 250mg. So you are trying to calculate how many or what portion of these vials you need to administer. You should be able to see immediately, though, that you will need more than one vial since one will only give 250mg. You can calculate this in different ways:

Logic

Each vial contains 250mg. If I give one vial that is 250 mg, this leaves 125mg still to give (375mg–250mg). 125mg is half of 250mg therefore I need to give one and a half of the vials.

Formula method

375mg (what you want to administer)
250mg (what you have available) =
3 (dividing top and bottom by 125)
2

= 1.5 ampoules

6. You need to administer ³/₄ of the available ampoule, as 15mg is ³/₄ of 20mg. This would be ³/₄ of 2ml, which is 1.5 ml (divide 2ml into 4 lots of 5ml parts). You could use any other method though to arrive at the answer of 1.5ml.

7. You first need to calculate the dose your patient requires which is 4mg x 45kg = 180mg (use a calculator or double 45mg twice, that is, 90mg and 90mg). You then need to calculate how many millilitres of 40mg/ml you need to administer. 180mg divided by

4 gives 160mg with 20mg left over. This would be 4 ampoules (4 x 40mg = 160mg) and then a half of an ampoule to give 20mg. You would need to administer 4.5 millilitres or 4 and a half ampoules. You could work this calculation out by any method to arrive at this answer. The method here, though, will help you to think about checking that your answer makes sense logically.

8. First, you need to convert 0.6mg so that it is in the same unit of measurement as the ampoule strength, that is, micrograms. To convert, you need to multiply 0.6mg by 1000 to get 600mcg. You now know you need to administer 600mcg and have ampoules that contain 400mcg. You could perhaps see logically that 600mcg is 400mcg plus 200mcg so you will need to administer 1.5 ampoules. Otherwise, use any method and consider the method here for checking your answer is logical.

9. First, you need to calculate the dose of vancomycin your patient needs according to their weight. This is 10mg x 15kg = 150mg. You then need to work out how much of the vial would contain this dose. Your reconstituted strength of vancomycin is 250mg/10ml. You could perhaps see now that 150mg is three-fifths of 250mg (dividing both into 50mg portions in your mind) so you will need ³/₅ of 10ml, which is 6ml. Use any method, though, to calculate that you need to administer 6ml here.

10. First, you need to convert 1.8g into milligrams so you can compare to the vial strength. This is 1.8g x 1000 = 1800mcg. You can then either divide 1800mg by 600mg (n.b. same as 18 divided by 6) or add 600mg together until you reach 1800mg. You would need to administer 3 vials.

CHAPTER 3

EXERCISE 22

1. 1000ml divided by 8 hours = 125ml/hr

2. 500ml divided by 8 hours = 63ml/hr (round up from 62.5ml)

3. 1000ml divided by 12 hours = 83ml/hr (round down from 83.3ml)

4. 500ml divided by 4 hours = 125ml/hr

5. 500ml divided by 6 hours = 83ml/hr (round down from 83.3ml)

EXERCISE 23

1. 33 dpm (rounding down from 33.3)

2. You need to administer 500ml 5% glucose to your patient over 6 hours. The manual giving set has a drop factor of 20. What rate would you set this infusion up for?

   (a) *Make sure you understand the question and what it is you are required to calculate:*

   I want my patient to have 500ml continuously over 6 hours. I am using a manual giving set so need to calculate the number of drops per minute to set the giving set up for.

   (b) *Write down the formula and ensure this is correct:*

   $$\frac{\text{volume to be infused (ml)}}{\text{duration (hours)}} \times \frac{\text{drop factor}}{60}$$
   = drips per minute (dpm)

   (c) *Extract the relevant numbers from practice and place into the formula:*

   $$\frac{500}{6} \times \frac{20}{60} = \text{drips per minute (dpm)}$$

   (d) *Chose the method you wish to use, that is, calculator or arithmetically:*

   Calculator

   $$\boxed{5}\,\boxed{0}\,\boxed{0}\,\boxed{\times}\,\boxed{2}\,\boxed{0}\,\boxed{\div}\,\boxed{6}\,\boxed{\div}\,\boxed{6}\,\boxed{0}\,\boxed{=}$$

Arithmetic

1) $\dfrac{10\,000}{360} = (\div 10)\ \dfrac{1000}{36}\ (\div 2) = \dfrac{500}{18}\ (\div 2) =$

$\dfrac{250}{9} = 9\overline{)250} =$

2) $\dfrac{500}{6}\ \dfrac{250}{3} \times \dfrac{1}{3}\ \dfrac{20}{60} = \dfrac{250}{9}$

(e) *Solve the calculation*

= 27.7′

(f) *Round your number up to the nearest whole number:*

   I would round this number up to 28 drops per minute.

(g) *Check your answer using a different method or repeating your calculation until you have a consistent numerical answer:*

   Use a different method from the one originally used above.

(h) *Using your knowledge of what it is you are trying to calculate place your numerical solution back into context, for example rate per hour or drips per minute:*

   I would use the regulator on the giving set to ensure that the speed of the drips would be 28 drops every minute.

(i) *Check that the answer you have obtained makes sense logically and using your clinical practice wexperience:*

   28 is a number I have seen before for drip rates.

(j) *Set manual giving set to the required drip rate per minute (that is, number of drips) and electronic device rate per hour (that is, number of millilitres per hour):*

I would approximate 28 to 30 drops per minute and estimate that I would need one drop for every two seconds. I would therefore manipulate the giving set regulator and count the drops going into the chamber until I had regulated it to approximately 30 drops every minute.

3. 31 dpm (rounding down from 31.25)

4. 42 dpm (rounding up from 41.6)

5. 28 dpm (rounding up 27.7)

EXERCISE 24

1. *Your patient has been prescribed 1000ml 0.9% sodium chloride over 8 hours. Using a manual giving set with a drop factor of 20 drops/ml, calculate the number of drops per minute you would set this infusion rate for.*

   Your calculation should have been $^{1000}\!/_8 \times {}^{20}\!/_{60}$ = 42 dpm (rounding up from 41.6)

2. *Your patient has been written up for a 1000ml infusion of 5% dextrose over 12 hours. What rate per hour would you set this infusion for using a volumetric pump?*

   Your calculation should have been $^{1000}\!/_{12}$ = 83ml/hr (rounding down from 83.3)

3. *You need to set up a unit of blood (500ml) for your patient to run over 2 hours. The giving set has a drop factor of 15 drops/ml. How many drips per minute would you set this infusion for?*

   Worked through answer:

   Your calculation would be:

   $$\frac{500ml}{2\ hours} \times \frac{15\ drops/ml}{60} = \frac{250}{1} \times \frac{1}{4} = \frac{125}{2} =$$
   62.5 which is 63 dpm (rounding up)

4. *The next IV infusion your patient has been written up for is now due and is 500ml dextrose saline over 6 hours.*

What rate per hour would you set for this infusion using a volumetric pump?

Your calculation would be 500ml/6 hours = 83ml/hr (rounding down from 83.3).

5. *Your colleague has set up a 1000ml infusion of 5% dextrose prescribed to run over 10 hours at a rate of 125ml/ hr. The infusion was commenced at 8am. What time would this infusion finish at this rate? Was this the correct rate?*

The infusion is running at 125ml every hour. At 125ml/hr the infusion would finish after 8 hours, which would be 4pm. This is 2 hours earlier than has been prescribed (10 hours after the infusion commenced at 8am should be 6pm). Therefore this was not the correct rate and it should have been set at a rate of 100ml/hr.

EXERCISE 25

1. 10g in 100ml

   100g in 1000ml

   Answer = 100g

2. 0.9g in 100ml

   To work out 500ml, either multiply 0.9 and 100ml by 5 or multiply by 10 to get the number of grams in 1000ml and then halve both to find out the number of grams in 500ml.

   Option 1   4.5g in 500ml
              (multiplying by 5)

   Option 2   9g in 1000ml
              (multiplying by 10)
              4.5g in 500ml (halving)
              Answer = 4.5g

3. 5g in 100ml

   Option 1   25g in 500ml
              (multiplying by 5)

   Option 2   50g in 1000ml
              (multiplying by 10)
              25g in 500ml (halving)
              Answer = 25g

EXERCISE 26

1. *Worked through answer:*

   $\dfrac{10}{100} \times 500 = 50g$

2. 9g

3. 20g

EXERCISE 27

1. *You need to set up an infusion of heparin 15 000 units over 24 hours. Calculate the amount of heparin required from the stock ampoules available of 25 000 units/1ml and the rate per hour for the syringe pump.*

   (a) *Ensure you understand what it is the question is asking you to calculate:*

   You need to ensure a continuous infusion of the drug prescribed over 24 hours.

   (b) *Calculate the amount of the ampoule(s) that contains the prescribed dosage:*

   I need 15 000 units and I have available 25 000 units. I can see that what I need is three-fifths of the 25 000 units so I need three-fifths of 1 ml, which is 0.6ml. Alternatively, I may use the formula and end up with ³/₅, which, I have learnt, is 0.6ml.

   (c) *Check that this amount makes sense logically and by using your practice experience:*

   The whole ampoule of 1ml would give 25 000 units and 0.5ml would give half of this, which is 12 500 units. 15 000 units would be between 0.5ml and 1ml, which is 0.6ml so this is a logical answer.

   (d) *Place this volume of the ampoule (s) into a 50ml syringe with a leur lock:*

   To do this you can use a needle and syringe and then add to the 50ml syringe.

   (e) *Draw up 0.9% sodium chloride into the syringe to give a total of 50ml:*

   Use a 100ml 0.9% sodium chloride infusion bag.

   (f) *Complete a label detailing contents of syringe and attach this to syringe:*

   This is important to document details of the syringe contents and infusion.

   (g) *Attach the infusion line and prime this:*

   Remember that priming will use approximately 2ml of the volume.

   (h) *Place syringe into the syringe pump and set rate for 2ml/hour:*

   The 48ml contain 15 000 units of heparin which will now infuse continuously over the 24-hour period.

2. *You need to set up an infusion containing 80mg dopamine hydrochloride in 50ml. The ampoules available are 40mg/ml. How many ampoules would you need?*

   You would need two dopamine ampoules of 40mg/1ml drawn up into a 50ml syringe and then the volume made up to 50ml with 0.9% sodium chloride.

3. *A patient requires a heparin infusion drawn up of 20 000 units in 50ml over 24 hours. The ampoules available are 25 000 units/ml. How many millilitres of the available ampoule will you need to draw up?*

   You will need ⁴/₅ of the ampoule, which is 0.8ml drawn up into a 50ml syringe and the volume made up to 50ml with 0.9% sodium chloride.

EXERCISE 28

1. *Worked though answer:*

    (a) 25mg in 50ml

        2.5mg in 5ml   divide by 10

        0.5 mg in 1ml   divide by 5

        Dosage in 1ml = 0.5mg

    (b) Infusion rate is 2ml/hr so
    2 x 0.5mg = 1mg

    Formula method

    $$\frac{25mg \times 2ml/hr}{50ml} = \frac{1}{2} \times 2 = 1mg$$

2. (a) = 1000 units in 1ml

    (b) = 4000 units

3. (a) = 1 unit

    (b) = 2 units

4. (a) = 600 units

    (b) = 1200 units

5. (a) = 1.6mg

    (b) = 3.2mg

EXERCISE 29

1. 3.9ml/hr

2. *Your patient needs to be administered 0.1mcg/kg/min of a drug. Your patient's weight is 70kg. The infusion used in your area is 12mg/50ml. Calculate the rate per hour you would set this infusion up for.*

    (a) *Ensure you understand what it is the question is asking you to calculate:*

    Need to calculate the rate per hour (ml/hr) required for an infusion.

    (b) *Calculate dose per weight of the patient: dosage/kg x patient's weight (kg):*

    0.1mcg x 70kg = 7mcg

    (c) *Multiply the dose for the patient per minute by 60 to work out dosage per hour for this patient:*

    7mcg x 60 = 420mcg

    (d) *Convert usual infusion dose into micrograms:*

    12mg x 1000 = 12 000mcg

    (e) *Caculate dosage per ml:*

    12 000mcg ÷ 50ml = 240mcg in 1ml

    (f) *Calculate ml/hr: dosage per hour ÷ dosage in 1ml:*

    420mg ÷ 240mg = 1.75ml/hr

    (g) *Check your answer by repeating calculation, using clinical experience or logic to ensure 100% certainty before administering drug.*

3. 1.8ml/hr

4. 5.85ml/hr or 5.9ml/hr rounded up to one decimal place

5. 3.24ml/hr or 3.2ml/hr rounded down to one decimal place

EXERCISE 30

1. Draw up 2 ampoules of morphine sulphate (60mg/ml), 1 ampoule of midazolam (10mg/2ml) and 2 ampoules of levomepromazine (25mg/1ml) into 10ml syringe and make volume up to length 48mm.

2. Draw up 1 ampoule of cyclizine (1ml) and half of the other ampoule (0.5ml) to give 1.5ml cyclizine (50mg/1ml). Draw up all of the morphine sulphate ampoule and two ampoules of haloperidol (5mg/1ml) using the same syringe and make volume up to length 48mm.

3. Draw up 1 ampoule of hyoscine hydrobromide (1ml) and half of the other ampoule (0.5ml) to give 1.5ml hyoscine hydrobromide (400mcg/1ml). 4 ampoules of morphine sulphate 60mg/ml) and 2 ampoules of midazolam (10mg/2ml) into a 20ml syringe. Make up the volume to length 48mm.

4. Draw up 0.5ml of the haloperidol (5mg/1ml) and 1ml morphine sulphate (30mg/ml) into a 10ml syringe and make up the volume to length 48mm.

5. *Worked through answer:*

   (a) *Ensure that you understand what it is you are calculating:*

   Need to add each of the required drugs into a 10ml syringe and make up the volume to a length of 48mm to put into a syringe driver.

   (b) *For each drug, calculate the required volume that contains the prescribed dose:*

   morphine sulphate: 3 x 60mg/2ml ampoule

   hyoscine butylbromide: 3 x 20mg/1ml ampoule

   (c) *Check that each calculation is correct through recalculating to check, clinical experience and logic:*

60mg + 60mg + 60mg = 180mg

20mg + 20mg + 20mg = 60mg

(d) *Draw up each drug either separately and add to a 10ml syringe or straight into a 20ml syringe:*

Draw up the hyoscine into a 20ml syringe and then draw up the morphine sulphate ampoules. Note that the volume required for the drugs will be 9ml in total. This volume will exceed the length of 48mm. A 20ml syringe will be required.

(e) *Make up the volume in the 20ml syringe by drawing up water for injection to a length of 48mm:*

Draw up water for injection into the 20 ml syringe so that the volume now measures 48mm.

(f) *Ensure that the syringe driver is an hourly syringe driver and that rate is set for 2mm/hr.*

Assessment 3 (Chapter 3)

1. *Using the IV medicine administration chart, calculate the infusion rate using a volumetric pump for the 0.9% sodium chloride.*

   1000ml over 8 hours = 1000/8 = 125ml/hr

2. *Using the IV medicine administration chart, calculate the drip rate for the blood transfusion (giving set drop factor of 15 drops/ml).*

   $\frac{500}{4} \times \frac{15}{60} = 125 \times \frac{1}{4} = 31$ dpm

   (rounded to nearest whole number)

3. *Using the IV medicine administration chart, calculate the number of grams of glucose in the dextrose saline infusion prescribed.*

   4% glucose = 4g in 100ml = 40g in 1000ml (multiplying both by 10) and 20mg in 500ml (dividing both by 2). The answer is 20mg.

4. *Your patient has been written up for the prescription below:*

Prescription		Stock ampoules available
morphine sulphate 60mg	administered over 24 hours via a syringe driver	morphine sulphate 60mg/2ml
midazolam 10mg		midazolam 10mg/2ml
levomepromazine 25mg		levomepromazine 25mg/1ml

Calculate the number of millilitres of the available stock ampoules for each drug. Using a 1-hour syringe driver, what rate (mm/hr) would you set this driver for?

Draw up half the ampoule of midazolam (10mg/2ml). 1ml morphine sulphate (60mg/ml) and 1ml levomepromzine (25mg/ml). Add all to 10ml syringe and make the volume up to length 48mm. With an hourly syringe driver, you need to set the rate so it runs a set amount every hour. Rate needs to be set to 2mm, which would be 2mm/hr for this syringe driver.

5. *You patient has been prescribed heparin 40 000 units/50ml over 24 hours. The stock ampoules of heparin available are 50 000 units/ml. How many millilitres of this ampoule would you need for the infusion? If you set this infusion rate as 2ml/hr, how many units of heparin would your patient be receiving every hour?*

Draw up four-fifths of the ampoule of heparin, which would be 0.8ml. 40 000 units in 50ml is the same as 800 units in 1ml (dividing both by 50), so 2ml will be 2 x 800 = 1600 units/hr.

6. *Your patient has been prescribed 1000ml 5% dextrose infusion over 12 hours. Using a manual giving set with a drop factor of 20 drops/ml, calculate what rate you would set this infusion for.*

Using the formula = 28 dpm (round to nearest whole number)

7. *Your patient needs to be administered 0.2mcg/kg/min of a drug. Your patient's weight is 65kg. The infusion used in your area is 12mg/50ml. Calculate the rate per hour you would set this infusion up for.*

Worked through answer:

what you want to give (dose for patient per hour) x volume it's in
what you have available (convert to same measurement as above)

$\frac{0.2\text{mcg} \times 65\text{kg} \times 60}{12\ 000\text{mcg}} \times 50\text{ml}$ = 3.3ml/hr (round up to one decimal place from 3.25)

8. *You set up an infusion of dopamine containing 80mg/50ml and set the rate as 3ml/hr. How many milligrams of the drug is the patient receiving per hour?*

Infusion contains 1.6mg/ml. Infusion is running at 3ml/hr so patient is receiving 1.6mg x 3 = 4.8mg/hr

9. *Your patient has been prescribed 50 units actrapid/50ml and requires 4 units per hour administered initially. What rate would you set this infusion for?*

4ml/hr

10. *You need to administer 1mcg/kg/min of a drug. The infusion available is 800mg/500ml and your patient weights 52kg. How many millilitres per hour would you set this infusion for?*

$\frac{1 \times 52 \times 60}{800\ 000} \times 500$ = 1.95ml/hr
(2ml/hr, rounded one decimal place)

CHAPTER 4

Test your maths skills

Question 1
(a) 625
(b) 270
(c) 187.5
(d) 1700
(e) 151

Question 2
(a) 250
(b) 500
(c) 1600
(d) 1000
(e) 1000

Question 3
(a) ¼
(b) ³⁄₈
(c) ¹⁄₁₆

(d) 2
(e) 62.5

Question 4
(a) 0.5
(b) 0.75
(c) 0.2
(d) 0.1
(e) 0.4

Question 5
(a) 100
(b) 62.5
(c) 20
(d) 215
(e) 1667

Question 6
(a) 100

(b) 50
(c) 50
(d) 30
(e) 9

Question 7
(a) 50 000
(b) 1800
(c) 125
(d) 5
(e) 0.3

Question 8
(a) 2000
(b) 900
(c) 25
(d) 99
(e) –10

Question 9
(a) 25ml
(b) ½
(c) 100ml
(d) 356ml
(e) 27mmHg

Question 10
(a) 1ml or half the
      ampoule
(b) 125ml/hr
(c) 0.5ml
(d) 3 ampoules
(e) 4 tablets

SESSION ONE – Maths Fitness

Times Table Answers

	1	2	3	4	5	6	7	8	9	10	11	12
1	1	2	3	4	5	6	7	8	9	10	11	12
2	2	4	6	8	10	12	14	16	18	20	22	24
3	3	6	9	12	15	18	21	24	27	30	33	36
4	4	8	12	16	20	24	28	32	36	40	44	48
5	5	10	15	20	25	30	35	40	45	50	55	60
6	6	12	18	24	30	36	42	48	54	60	66	72
7	7	14	21	28	35	42	49	56	63	70	77	84
8	8	16	24	32	40	48	56	64	72	80	88	96
9	9	18	27	36	45	54	63	72	81	90	99	108
10	10	20	30	40	50	60	70	80	90	100	110	120
11	11	22	33	44	55	66	77	88	99	110	121	132
12	12	24	36	48	60	72	84	96	108	120	132	144

EXERCISE 31

1. 10
2. 100
3. 1000
4. 60
5. 1250

6. 0.1
7. 1
8. 10
9. 7
10. 100

EXERCISE 32

Question	ten thousands	thousands	hundreds	tens	units	tenths	hundredths	thousandths
1			1	7	5			
2					1	4		
3				3	7			
4					0	1	2	5
5		1	0	0	0	2	5	

Assessment for Session One

1. 2   10   25
2. 10 parts
3. 3 places
4. 8 = tens, 7 = units and 5 = tenths
5. 1000
6. 15
7. 125
8. 1.8
9. 0.5
10. 62.5

SESSION TWO – Maths Stamina

EXERCISE 33

1. 10 x 1000 = 10 000
2. 0.004 x 100 = 0.4
3. 0.7 ÷ 10 = 0.07
4. 0.0125 x 1000 = 12.5
5. 50 ÷ 100 = 0.5

EXERCISE 34

1.
$$\begin{array}{r} 0\ 2\ 7.7\ 7' \\ 9\overline{\smash{\big)}2\ {}_{2}5\ 70.\ 70\ 0} \end{array}$$

2.
$$\begin{array}{r} 0.\ 3\ 7\ 5 \\ 8\overline{\smash{\big)}3.\ {}_{3}0\ {}_{6}0\ {}_{4}0} \end{array}$$

3.
$$\begin{array}{r} 0\ 2\ 0\ 0 \\ 5\overline{\smash{\big)}1\ {}_{1}0\ 0\ 0} \end{array}$$

4.
$$\begin{array}{r} 1\ 5\ 0 \\ 5\overline{\smash{\big)}7\ {}_{2}5\ 0.\ 0\ 0} \end{array}$$

5.
$$\begin{array}{r} 1\ 6\ 8.\ 7\ 5 \\ 4\overline{\smash{\big)}6\ {}_{2}7\ {}_{3}5.\ {}_{3}0\ {}_{2}0} \end{array}$$

EXERCISE 35

1. *Give two equivalent fractions for* $^4/_{12}$
   $^1/_3$ or $^2/_6$ or $^8/_{24}$ or $^{16}/_{48}$ and so on
2. *Express* $^3/_4$ *in two different ways*
   $^9/_{12}$ or $^6/_8$ or $^{12}/_{16}$ and so on or as a
   decimal 0.75

3. *Express ½ in four different ways*

   ²/4 or ⁴/8 or ⁸/16 or ¹²/24 or ⁵/10 or ⁹/18 and so on, or as a decimal 0.5

4. *Give an equivalent fraction for ²⁵/100*

   Divide both top and bottom by 5 to get ⁵/20 and then both by 5 again to get ¼. Or you could divide both 25 and 100 by 25 to get ¼

5. *Give an equivalent fraction for ⁴⁹/84*

   This is where your knowledge of times tables comes in useful! If you had revised this, then you should see that both top and bottom are divisible by 7 to give you ⁷/12.

EXERCISE 36

1. *What is the lowest equivalent fraction of ¹²⁵/500?*

   Divide top and bottom numbers by 5 to get ²⁵/100, and again to get ⁵/20 and again to get ¼. Or if you could have divided top and bottom by 25 or by 125 if you recognised that 500 is divisible by 125.

2. *What is the lowest equivalent fraction of ⁵⁰⁰/750?*

   Divide top and bottom numbers by 250 to get ²/3.

3. *Express ²/10 as a decimal and give the lowest equivalent fraction*

   ²/10 is 0.2. You can calculate this by dividing 2 by 10 and moving the decimal point one place. The lowest equivalent fraction is ⅕ (dividing top and bottom numbers by 2).

4. *Express 0.6 as a fraction and give another equivalent fraction for this*

   0.6 is six-tenths using the number line. This is expressed as ⁶/10. Another equivalent fraction can be found by dividing top and bottom numbers by 2 to get ³/5.

5. *Express 0.75 as a fraction*

   You should be able to recognise that this is the same as ⁷⁵/100, which you can reduce down to ³/4 by dividing top and bottom numbers by 25.

EXERCISE 37

1. $\frac{1}{3} \times \frac{1}{2} = \frac{1 \times 1}{3 \times 2} = \frac{1}{6}$

2. $\frac{1}{8} \times \frac{1}{2} = \frac{1 \times 1}{8 \times 2} = \frac{1}{16}$

3. $\frac{2}{5} \times \frac{1}{4} = \frac{2 \times 1}{5 \times 4} = \frac{2}{20}$ or $\frac{1}{10}$

4. $\frac{3}{4} \times \frac{1}{2} = \frac{3 \times 1}{4 \times 2} = \frac{3}{8}$

5. $\frac{1}{8} \times \frac{4}{5} = \frac{1 \times 4}{8 \times 5} = \frac{4}{40} = \frac{1}{10}$

EXERCISE 38

1. 5
2. 3
3. 4
4. 3
5. 10

EXERCISE 39

1. $\frac{1}{4} \div \frac{1}{6} = \frac{1}{4} \times 6 = \frac{6}{4} = \frac{3}{2}$
2. $2 \div \frac{1}{5} = 2 \times 5 = 10$
3. $\frac{1}{3} \div \frac{1}{6} = \frac{1}{3} \times 6 = \frac{6}{3} = 2$
4. $4 \div \frac{1}{8} = 4 \times 8 = 32$
5. $\frac{2}{5} \div \frac{1}{10} = \frac{2}{5} \times \frac{10}{1} = \frac{20}{5} = 4$

EXERCISE 40

1. $\frac{1}{2} + \frac{1}{3} = \frac{5}{6}$
2. $\frac{3}{4} + \frac{1}{2} = 1\frac{1}{4}$
3. $\frac{3}{5} - \frac{1}{5} = \frac{2}{5}$

4. $^1/8 + ^1/2 = {}^5/8$

5. *Worked through answer:*

   Common denominator is 40:

   Stage 1

   $^2/5 - ^3/8$ = $\dfrac{16 -}{40}$

   5 into 40 = 8

   8 x 2 = 16

   Stage 2

   $^2/5 - ^3/8$ = $\dfrac{16 - 15}{40}$

   8 into 40 = 5

   5 x 3 = 15

   Subtract the top numbers:

   $\dfrac{16 - 15}{40}$ = $\dfrac{1}{40}$

Assessment for Session Two

1. $^1/2$

2. $^1/8 = 8 \overline{\smash{\big)}\,1.\,10\ 20\ 40}$ ⟶ $0.\ 1\ 2\ 5$

3. 100

4. $1000 \times \dfrac{20}{8} = 125 \times ^1/3 = \dfrac{125}{3} = 3\overline{\smash{\big)}\,1\ 12\ 5.\ 20\ 20}$ ⟶ $0\ 41.\ 6\ 6$

   = 41.66′ (the number 6 will continue recurring for infinity! We represent this mathematically with an apostrophe)

5. $^{20}/50 \times 2 = ^2/5 \times 2 = ^4/5 = 0.8$

6. $^1/4 \div ^1/8 = = ^1/4 \times ^8/1 = ^8/4 = 2$

7. $^1/5 + ^2/3 = \dfrac{(3 \times 1) + (5 \times 2)}{15} = \dfrac{3 + 10}{15} = {}^{13}/15$

8. $^1/2 - ^1/8 = \dfrac{(4 \times 1) - (1 \times 1)}{8} = \dfrac{4 - 1}{8} = {}^3/8$

9. 5mg is one quarter of 20mg therefore you need to administer one quarter of 2ml. This is $^1/4 \times 2 = ^2/4 = ^1/2 = 0.5$ml. Or you could use the formula of $^5/20 \times 2 = ^1/4 \times 2 = ^2/4 = ^1/2 = 0.5$ml.

10. You could work out that 60mg is four times 15mg so you need to administer 4 x 2ml = 8ml. Or you could use the formula of $^{60}/15 \times 2 = 4 \times 2 = 8$ml.

SESSION THREE – How supple are you?

EXERCISE 41

1. 15g out of 100g = 15%

2. 75ml out of 100ml = 75%

3. 40 sweets out of 100 sweets = 40%

4. 25 donkeys out of 100 donkeys = 25%

5. 10mcg out of 100mcg = 10%

EXERCISE 42

1. 10% of 164 = $^{10}/100$ of 164 = $^{10}/100 \times 164 = ^1/10 \times 164 = 16.4$ (this is the same as dividing by 10 and therefore moving the decimal point one place to the left)

2. 5% of 1000 = $^5/100$ of 1000 = $^5/100 \times 1000 = ^1/20 \times 1000 = 50$

3. 72% of 36 = $^{72}/100$ of 36 = $^{72}/100 \times 36 = ^{18}/25 \times 36 = 25.92$ (I found it helpful to use a calculator here, but you could do it using long multiplication and long division!!)

4. 2% of 48 = $^2/100$ of 48 = $^2/100 \times 48 = ^1/20 \times 48 = 0.96$ (calculator used here too!)

5. 0.9% of 1000 = $^{0.9}/100$ of 1000 = $^{0.9}/100 \times 1000 = 0.9 \times 10 = 9$

EXERCISE 43

1. The question is asking how many grams of glucose are there in a 1000ml infusion bag if 5% is 5g in 100ml? Remember that 5% is saying 5 for every 100. So in this case it is saying 5g of glucose is dissolved in

every 100ml. If you take 10 times this amount of fluid, that is, 1000ml, then there must be 10 times the amount of glucose, that is, 10 x 5 = 50g. Alternatively, you could calculate $^5/_{100}$ x 1000 = 50g.

2. The question is asking how many grams of sodium chloride there are in a 1000ml infusion bag if 0.9% means 0.9g in 100ml. Remember that 0.9% is saying 0.9 for every 100. So in this case it is saying 0.9g of sodium chloride is dissolved in every 100ml. If you take ten times this amount of fluid, that is, 1000ml then there must be ten times the amount of sodium chloride ie 10x 0.9 = 9g. Alternatively you could calculate $^{0.9}/_{100}$ x 1000 = 9g.

EXERCISE 44

	Percentages	Fractions	Decimals
1.	10%	$^1/_{10}$	0.1
2.	33.3′%	$^3/_{10}$	0.33′
3.	12.5%	$^1/_8$	0.125
4.	50%	$^1/_2$	0.5
5.	75% and 25%	$^3/_4$ and $^1/_4$	0.75 and 0.25
6.	25%	$^1/_4$	0.25

EXERCISE 45

1. 74%

2. 8.2% (rounding up from 8.15)

3. 30%

4. 70%

5. 92%

EXERCISE 46

1. $^4/_{72}$ x 100 = 5.6% (rounding up from 5.56)

2. $^{800}/_{1000}$ x 100 = 80%

3. $^{15}/_{100}$ x 110 = 16.5. 110 – 16.5 = 93.5 or 94 rounding up bpm (beats per minute)

4. $^{30}/_{100}$ x 20 = 6 20 + 6 = 26

5. $^{25}/_{100}$ x 40 = 10. 40 + 10 = 50m

Assessment for Session Three

1.

Fractions	Decimals	Percentages
$^1/_2$	0.5	50%
$^3/_5$	0.6	60%
$^1/_4$	0.25	25%
$^3/_4$	0.75	75%
$^1/_5$	0.2	20%

2. $^{15}/_{25}$ x 100 = $^3/_5$ x 100 = $^{300}/_5$ = 60%

3. $^{25}/_{125}$ x 100 = $^1/_5$ x 100 = $^{100}/_5$ = 20%

4. $^{25}/_{100}$ = 0.25

5. You have reduced the tablets by 5 (20 – 15 = 5). You need to work out percentage of 5 out of 20 = $^5/_{20}$ x 100 = $^1/_4$ x 100 = 25%

6. 5% = $^5/_{100}$ x 1000 = 50g. Or you could work out that 5% = 5 out of 100 so would be 10 times this amount for 1000 = 50g

7. You need to work out 10% of current dose and then add this to the current dose. 10% = $^{10}/_{100}$ x 20 = $^1/_{10}$ x 20 = 2mg. 20mg + 2mg = 22mg.

8. $^{25}/_{100}$ x 1000 = $^1/_4$ x 1000 = 250

9. Your patient has received 200 out of 500 = $^{200}/_{500}$ x 100 = $^2/_5$ x 100 = 40%

10. You need to work out the reduction in admissions and then calculate the percentage of this to the original admission figure: 1250 – 1200 – 50. The admissions have reduced by 50. $^{50}/_{1250}$ x 100 = $^2/_5$ x 10 = $^{20}/_5$ = 4%. Your hospital has not met its target for this month!

SESSION FOUR – Through the Pain Barrier!

EXERCISE 47

1. 4

2. 1. The fraction is $\frac{1}{10}$

3. 1g. The fraction is $\frac{1}{1000}$

EXERCISE 48

1. Half is the same as saying that Jack gets 1 out of 2 questions right, which is 1:2

2. 1:6 (dividing both sides by 4)

3. What do you have to do to 1000ml to get to 1ml? You need to divide by 1000. Therefore you need to divide the other side of the ratio by the same amount to get 1mg.

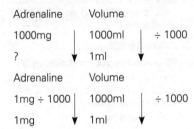

Adrenaline	Volume	
1000mg	1000ml	÷ 1000
?	1ml	
Adrenaline	Volume	
1mg ÷ 1000	1000ml	÷ 1000
1mg	1ml	

Assessment for Session Four

1. 5 chocolates each!

2. 50 patients

3. 2:1

4. The ratio is 2 staff:12 patients. 36 patients is three times 12, so you need 3 x the number of staff, which is 2 x 3 = 6 staff.

5. *The strength of an adrenaline ampoule (1ml) is 1:1000 (g:ml). If you administer 3 ampoules of this adrenaline how many milligrams have you administered? (1g = 1000mg):*

1:1000 = 1g:1000ml = 1000mg:1000ml = 1mg:1ml. Administering 3 ampoules of 1ml each would be 3mg.

6. You need to give three lots of 10mg to give 30mg so you need three lots of 2ml which is 3 x 2ml = 6ml.

7. *The dose of an adrenaline ampoule is 1:1000 (g:ml). How many milligrams in 1ml? (Note that I am asking for your answer to be in milligrams – n.b. 1g = 1000mg):*

1:1000 = 1g:1000ml = 1000mg:1000ml = 1mg:1ml. Therefore 1mg in 1ml.

8. You need ten times the volume to dilute with, which is 10 x 10ml = 100ml.

9. *The adrenaline ampoule strength is 1:100 (g:ml). Express this ratio in milligrams (n.b. 1 mg = 1000mg):*

1:100 = 1g:100ml = 1000mg:100ml = 10mg:1ml

10. *Express the adrenaline 1:1000 (g:ml) strength in the ratio of milligrams to millilitres:*

1:1000 = 1g:1000ml = 1000mg:1000ml = 1mg:1ml.

SESSION FIVE – Running the 5K Maths Challenge!

Lap 1

1. Your calculation should have been $\frac{20}{50}$ x 2 = 0.8 ml

Lap 2

1. Diclofenac tablets are 25mg. As you need 50mg, you will need two of these tablets.

2. Paracetamol tablets are 500mg. You need to convert the prescribed dose to milligrams. To convert grams to milligrams you need to multiply by 1000 to give 1000mg. As you need 1000mg you will need two of these tablets.

Lap 3

1. Your calculation should have been $^{15\,000}/_{25\,000} \times 1$. This would give you 0.6ml. If you've done this another way, this is also fine. For example, you may have 'seen' that 15 000 is $^3/_5$ of 25 000 and knew that $^3/_5$ of 1 is 0.6ml.

Lap 4

1. If you need 50ml and the heparin makes up 0.6ml of this, the remainder would be 50 – subtract 0.6 to give 49.4ml!

Lap 5

1. A ratio of 10mg/5ml is the same as 20 mg/10ml (always 'doing the same' to both the volume and the weight, that is, in this case, doubling). You would administer 10ml of oramorph to Jessica.

Lap 6

1. Your calculation should have two stages. First, work out 50% of 20mg and second, add this to 20mg to get the new dose:

   (a) $^{50}/_{100} \times 20$ will give you 50% of 20 = 10

   (b) 20 + 10 = 30

Jessica's new dose is therefore 30mg oramorph.

Lap 7

Convert 0.25mg to micrograms by multiplying by 1000. This gives 125 mcg tablets.

1. Mr Chandra would need 2 of these tablets to give 250mcg (two lots of 125mcg gives 250mcg)

2. 4 tablets would give 125 x 4 = 500mcg or 0.5mg (so you would need to clarify with Mr Chandra's GP or pharmacist!)

Lap 8

1. Your calculation should be $^{1000}/_8 \times ^{20}/_{60} = 41.66'$. Therefore would be 42 drips per minute

Lap 9

5% dextrose means 5g out of every 100ml. Therefore your calculation should have been $^5/_{100} \times 1000 = 50$g dextrose

Lap 10

Your calculation should be $^{1000}/_8 = 125$ ml/hr

Lap 11

There are 30 patients on Baldrick ward: 20% of these patients have pressure sores, 80% have IVs running and 50% have been prescribed laxatives. Work out the number of patients:

1. *With pressure sores:*

   20 divided by 100 multiplied by 30 gives the answer of 6 patients. Alternatively, you could know that 20% is one-fifth and work out a fifth of 30 to be 6.

2. *Who have IVs:*

   80 divided by 100 multiplied by 30 gives 24 patients. Or, as before, you could recognise that 80% is four-fifths and work out a fifth of 30 and multiply this by 4.

3. *Who have been prescribed laxatives:*

   50 divided by 100 and multiplied by 30 will give 15 patients

Lap 12

1:6 means that for every 6 patients there is one staff member. For two staff, there would be 12 patients, 3 staff would have 18 patients, 4 staff would have 24 patients and 5 staff would have 30 patients. Therefore 5 staff work on an early shift on Baldrick ward. Another, simpler, way of working this out is by dividing the 30 patients by 6 to get 5 staff.

CHAPTER 5

Assessment 1

1. 2 vials

2. 2 tablets

3. First, convert the prescribed dose to micrograms by multiplying 0.25 by 1000; 0.25 x 1000 = 250. 125mcg and 125mcg gives 250mcg so the answer is 2 tablets.

4. Calculate the dose required for this baby by multiplying dose/kg by the baby's weight; 7.5mg x 5.4kg = 40.5mg.

5. 3 tablets

6. Divide 375mg by 3 to get 125mg.

7. Multiply dose/kg by the weight of the child; 2mg x 19 = 38mg.

8. Divide 30mg by 3 to get the milligram strength of each dose = 10mg. The tablets are 5mg so you would need to administer 2 tablets.

9. First, convert the prescribed dose to milligrams; 0.45 x 1000 = 450mg. Divide this dose by 3 to get the strength required for each dose = 150mg. The tablets available are 100mg and 50mg so you would need to give one tablet of each.

10. Adrenaline 1:1000 = 1g:1000ml. Convert 1g into milligrams by multiplying by 1000 = 1000mg: 1000ml. Divide each side by 1000 to find the milligram strength of 1ml = 1mg.

11. Calculate dose of gentamicin by multiplying dose/kg by Davy's weight; 2mg x 60 = 120mg.

12. The ampoules are 40mg/ml so you would need 3 ampoules to make up a 120mg strength (40 + 40 + 40 = 120).

13. Davy requires 60mg morphine. The ampoules available are 30mg/ml so you would need to administer 2 ampoules (30 x 2 = 60).

14. 4 x 62.5mcg = 250mcg. The prescribed dose is 500mcg so your colleague has not prepared the right number of tablets. For this tablet strength, you need 8 tablets (n.b. as this is a large number you may need to check the availability of a 125mcg or 250mcg tablet strength). You also need to follow the procedures in your area for a near-miss drug error.

15. The adrenaline strength is 1:1000 in 1ml ampoule. Remember that this means 1g:1000ml. Convert the grams to milligrams to get 1000mg:1000ml and divide both sides by 1000 to get 1mg:1ml. To administer 6mg, you would need to give 6 ampoules.

16. First, calculate the total daily dose by multiplying dose/kg by patient's weight; 50mg x 30 = 1500mg. This needs to be administered in three divided dosages so divide by 3 to get 500mg. The capsules available are 250mg so you would need to give two capsules (250mg + 250mg = 500mg).

17. First, calculate the total daily dose by multiplying dose/kg by patient's weight; 3mg x 25 = 75mg. This needs to be administered in three divided dosages so divide by 3 to get 25mg. The tablets available are 25mg so you would need to give 1 tablet.

18. 6 tablets of prednisolone 5mg would be 6 x 5 = 30mg. The prescription is for 25mg so your colleague has made an error. The correct number of tablets should be 5. You also need to follow the procedures in your area for a near miss drug error.

19. 500mg divided by 2 would give 250mg per dose. The suppositories contain 125mg so you would need to administer 2 (125mg + 125mg = 250mg).

20. Convert 3g into milligrams to give 3000 milligrams. The capsules contain 250mg. 3000 ÷ 250 = 12 capsules (n.b. this is a large number of capsules and also an unusually high dose for amoxicillin. You would need to check this with the prescriber and/or pharmacist).

Assessment 2

1. Adrenaline 1:100 means 1g:100ml. Convert 1g to milligrams to get 1000mg:100ml. Divide both sides by 100 to work out milligram strength in 1ml = 10mg.

2. Calculate daily dosage by multiplying dose/kg by patient's weight; 300mg x 12 = 3600mg. Divide this by 4 to give the individual dose 900mg.

3. 2 tablets

4. Convert prescribed dose to micrograms; 0.6 x 1000 = 600mg. The available ampoules are 400mcg. You can either 'see' that you need 1 ampoule and 1 half ampoule or use the formula $^{600}/_{400}$ x 1 = 1.5ml.

5. The individual dose is 240mg divided by 4 = 60mg. The tablets available are 30mg so you would need to give 2 tablets.

6. The prescription is for 300mg and the tablets available are 100mg so you should administer 100mg + 100mg + 100mg = 300mg = 3 tablets. Your colleague has made a near-miss drug error and you need to follow the procedure for your clinical area in reporting this.

7. Calculate the total dose for the patient by multiplying dose/kg by patient's weight; 100mg x 4 = 400mg.

8. Calculate the total dose for the patient by multiplying dose/kg by patient's weight; 1mg x 75 = 75mg. The tablets are 25mg so you would need to administer 3 tablets.

9. Calculate the total daily dose for the patient by multiplying dose/kg by patient's weight; 60mg x 22 = 1320mg. Divide this by 3 to get the individual dose = 440mg.

10. 2g = 2000mg. Therefore administer 4 tablets (500mg + 500mg + 500mg + 500mg = 2000mg).

11. Cefpodixime and phenytoin

12. 10ml

13. 5ml

14. 5ml

15. Calculate the total daily dose by multiplying dose/kg by the baby's weight; 40mg x 5 = 200mg. Divide by 4 to get the individual dose of 50mg.

16. Adrenaline 1:1000 means 1g:1000ml. Convert 1g to milligrams to give 1000mg:1000ml. Divide both sides by 1000 to give 1mg:1ml. You would need to administer 4 ampoules, that is, 4 ml.

17. 4 x 250mg = 1g. The prescription is for 1g so your colleague has prepared the right dose.

18. Calculate the total daily dose by multiplying dose/kg by the patient's weight; 25mg x 7.8 = 195mg. Divide by 3 to get the individual dose = 65mg.

19. Calculate the total daily dose for the patient by multiplying dose/kg by the patient's weight; 4mg x 37.5 = 150mg. Divide by 2 to get the individual dose of 75mg. You would need to administer one 50mg tablet and one 25mg tablet or 3 of the 25mg tablets.

20. 3g divided by 3 gives 1g three times a day. The tablets are 500mg so you would need to give 2 tablets.

Assessment 3

1. 2.5ml

2. 10ml

3. 1.5ml

4. Calculate the total daily dose = 50mg x 18kg = 900. Divide by 3 to get the individual doses = 300mg. You need to administer 6ml of the suspension.

5. The total dose required is 2mg x 78kg = 156mg. You need to administer 3.9ml.

6. The total dose required is 25mg x 3kg = 75mg. You need to add 10ml – 0.5ml (displacement volume) = 9.5ml. You now have a solution 600mg/10ml. You need to administer 1.25ml.

7. 10ml

8. 60ml

9. Calculate the total daily dosage 36mg x 26kg = 936mg. Divide by 2 to get the individual dose of 468mg. You can then work out the amount to administer = 9.75ml.

10. 3ml or 3 ampoules

11. Clarithromycin and paracetamol

12. 7.5ml

13. 25mg x 18kg = 450mg. Administer 0.75ml.

14. 1ml syringe

15. 10ml

16. 7.5ml

17. Should administer 0.5ml. Your colleague has prepared the correct amount.

18. 25ml

19. 4 ampoules

20. Adrenaline 1:100 means 1g:100ml. Convert 1g to milligrams = 1000mg:100ml. Divide both sides by 1000 to find out how many milligrams in 1ml = 10mg. You need to administer 5mg so you need to give 0.5ml.

Assessment 4

1. 20ml

2. 2mg x 72 = 144mg. You need to administer 3.6ml.

3. 30ml

4. Adrenaline 1:100 means 1g:100ml. Convert 1g to milligrams = 1000mg:100ml. Divide both sides by 1000 to give 10mg:1ml. You need to administer 0.6ml.

5. You need to add water for injection 5ml – 0.2ml (displacement volume) = 4.8ml. You will make a solution 250mg/5ml. You need to administer 1.25ml.

6. Total dose = 250mcg x 12kg = 3000mcg. Convert to milligrams = 3mg. You need to administer 3ml.

7. 0.4ml

8. 25ml

9. Your colleague has prepared 125mg x 4 = 500mg. The prescribed dose is 1g so your colleague has made an error. You need to follow the procedure for your clinical area to report near-miss drug errors.

10. 10ml

11. Sodium valporate and morphine sulphate

12. 0.25ml

13. 20mg x 15.6kg = 312mg. Sodium valporate strength 400mg/4ml. Administer 3.12ml.

14. 1ml

15. 200mcg x 9.8kg = 1960mcg. Convert to milligrams = 1.96mg. Administer 1.96ml.

16. 1.5ml or one and a half ampoules

17. The patient has been given 10ml of 125mg/5ml = 250mg. This is the correct dosage.

18. 50mg x 1.2kg = 60mg. Divided by 4 gives the dose of 15mg four times a day. You would add 5ml – 0.4ml (displacement volume) = 4.6ml to give a solution of 600mg/5ml. You would administer 0.125ml.

19. 0.85ml

20. 5mg x 14.8kg = 74mg. You make a solution of vancomycin 125mg/10ml and would administer 5.92ml.

Assessment 5

1. $^{1000}/8$ = 125ml/hr

2. $^{500}/6$ = 83.3ml/hr

3. 28 dpm (rounding up from 27.7')

4. 42 dpm (rounding up from 41.6')

5. 28 dpm (rounding up from 27.7')

6. 20g glucose

7. 9g

8. You would need 0.6ml of heparin (50 000 units/ml). The infusion would contain 30 000/50ml. This would be 600 units per ml (30 000/50) and therefore 2400 units per ml.

9. 80mg/50ml = 1.6mg/1ml. A rate of 5ml/hr = 5 x 1.6mg = 8mg per hour.

10. $\underline{\text{0.2mcg x 55kg x 60}}$ x 50ml = 2.8ml/hr
    12 000mcg
    (rounded to one decimal place)

11. 2ml

12. 50 units/50ml = 1unit/hr so your 2units would be 2ml/hour

13. $\underline{\text{1mcg x 67kg x 60}}$ x 500ml = 2.5
    800 000mcg
    (to one decimal place)

14. morphine (60mg/2ml) = 2ml
    midazolam (10mg/2ml) = 2ml
    levomepromazine (25mg/1ml) = 1ml
    Make up the volume to a length of 48mm. Set rate for 2mm/hr.

15. Patient requires 500mcg x 57kg per hour = 28 500mcg. Converted to milligrams = 28.5mg/hr. The infusion strength is 500mg/500ml = 1mg/1ml. So rate = 28.5ml/hr.

16. 100 units x 50kg = 5000 units/hr x 24 = 120 000 units

    The available ampoules are 50 000units/ml = $^{120\,000}/50\,000$ x 1 = 2.4ml

17. $\underline{\text{5mcg x 28kg x 60}}$ x 50ml = 5.3
    80 000
    (rounded to one decimal place)

18. morphine sulphate (60mg/1ml) = 4ml
    hyoscine butylbromide (400mcg/1ml) = 1.5ml
    midazolam (10mg/2ml) = 1ml
    Total volume 6.5ml. You would need a 20ml syringe and make up the volume to length 48mm with water for injection. Set driver for 2mm/hr.

19. 50mg x 1.2kg = 60mg. Each dose is 60 divided by 4 = 15mg. You would make up the 250mg vial using 10ml – 0.2ml (displacement volume) = 9.8ml to make 250mg/10ml. Administer 0.6ml.

20. Patient requires 500mcg x 35kg per hour = 17500mcg. Converted to milligrams = 17.5mg/hr. The infusion strength is 500mg/500ml = 1mg/1ml. So rate = 17.5ml/hr.

Assessment 6

1. $^{1000}/8$ = 125ml/hr

2. $^{500}/6$ = 83.3ml/hr

3. Add 1ml potassium (20mmol/10ml).
$^{100}/4$ = 25ml/hr (n.b. you could also
calculate $^{101}/4$ = 25.3ml/hr but the
difference is negligible)

4. 63 dpm (rounding up from 62.5 dpm)

5. 31 dpm (rounding down from 31.25)

6. 25g

7. 21 dpm (rounding up from 20.8 dpm)

8. 20g

9. 50 units/50ml = 1unit/1ml. 3ml/hr =
3 units

10. Infusion needs to be set for 2ml/hr
(n.b. 2ml used to prime infusion line).
Patient would receive 1000 units/hr.

11. Patient requires 500mcg x 75.8kg
per hour = 28900mcg. Converted to
milligrams = 28.9mg/hr. The infusion
strength is 500mg/500ml =
1mg/1ml. So rate = 28.9ml/hr.

12. 50 000 units/50ml = 48 000
units/48ml = 1000 units/ml. The
patient requires 4000 units/ml/hr so
would need the rate of 4ml/hr. Your
colleague is correct.

13. morphine sulphate (60mg/1ml) = 2ml
hyoscine butylbromide (400mcg/1ml)
= 1.5ml
clonazepam (1mg/1ml) = 1ml
Total volume = 4.5ml. Make up the
volume to length 48mm using water
for injection. Set the driver for 2mm/hr.

14. Patient requires 5mcg x 35.8kg x 60
= rate per person per hour =
10740mcg. Convert to milligrams =
10.74. Rate per ml = $^{80}/50$ = 1.6mg/
ml. Divide 10.74 by 1.6 = 6.7ml/hr.

15. Calculate rate for this person =
0.4mcg x 35.5kg = 18.2mcg.
Multiply this by 60 to work out dose
per hour so 18.2mcg x 60 = 852mcg.
Convert to milligrams = 0.852mg.
Calculate milligrams in 1ml = $^{12}/50$ =
0.24. Divide rate for person in hours

by dose per ml = 0.852 ÷ 0.24 =
3.55 or 3.6ml/hr (rounding up).

16. Prescription for aminophylline is
500mcg x 77.8/hour = 38900mcg/hr.
Convert this dose to milligrams =
38.9mg/hr. The infusion is
500mg/500ml = 1mg/ml. You would
need to set the infusion for 38.9ml/hr.
Your colleague is not correct and you
need to follow the procedure in your
clinical area for near-miss drug errors.

17. 50mg x 0.8mg = 40mg total daily
dose and divided by 4 gives dose
four times a day = 10mg. The 250mg
vial needs to be reconstituted with
10mg – 0.2ml (displacement volume)
= 9.8ml to make a solution of
250mg/10ml. You would need to
administer 0.4ml.

18. morphine sulphate (60mg/1ml) = 4ml
haloperidol (5mg/1ml) = 0.3ml
hyoscine butylbromide (400mcg/1ml)
= 0.5ml
Total volume = 4.8ml. Make this
volume up to length 48mm and set
the driver for 2mm/hr.

19. 2mcg x 16.8kg x $^{60}/80 000$ x 50 = 1.26
or 1.27ml/hr (rounding up) or rate per
hour for patient = 2mcg x 16.8 =
33.6mcg. Multiply by 60 to get per
hour = 2016. Convert to milligrams =
2.016mg. Divide this by amount per
ml = $^{80}/50$ =1.6mg. 2.016/1.6mg =
1.26 or 1.3ml/hr (round up).

20. A blood glucose reading of
15.2mmols/L = 4 units/hr = 4ml/hr

Assessment 7

1. 2 ampoules

2. 1.5ml

3. 2 tablets

4. 20ml

5. 125ml/hr

6. 100ml/hr

7. 83ml/hr (rounding down from 83.3)

8. 40g glucose and 1.8g sodium chloride

9. 500mcg x 56.7kg = 28350. Convert to milligrams = 28.35mg. 500mg/500ml infusion = 1mg/1ml. Infusion rate = 28.4mg (rounding up from 28.35)

10. 7.5mg x 5.2kg = 39mg. You need to administer 1.56ml.

11. 10mg x 12.5kg = 125mg. The vial needs reconstituting with 10ml – 0.4ml (displacement volume) = 9.6ml to make a solution of 250mg/10ml. You need to administer 5ml.

12. 5ml

13. 0.4ml

14. 10ml

15. Flucloxacillin and morphine sulphate

16. Adrenaline 1:100 means 1g:100ml. Convert to milligrams = 1000mg:100ml, dividing by 1000 = 10mg:1ml. You need to administer 0.8ml.

17. 125mg

18. 33 dpm (rounding down from 33.3')

19. 2mcg x 50.8kg x $^{60}/_{80\,000}$ x 50 = 3.81 or 3.8ml/hr (rounding down). Alternatively, you could calculate rate per hour for patient as 2 x 50.8 x 60 = 6.096mcg. Convert to milligrams = 6.096. Work rate per ml as $^{80}/_{50}$ = 1.6mg/ml. Divide rate per hour by rate per ml = 6.096/1.6 = 3.81 or 3.8ml/hr.

20. 25 000 units/50ml = 500 units/1ml. 2ml/hr = 1000 units. Yes, this is the correct rate.

Assessment 8

1. 2 tablets

2. 20ml

3. 2.5ml

4. 100mg/5ml so 400mg/20ml (multiplying both sides by 4)

5. 200mg twice daily

6. morphine sulphate (60mg/ml) = 6ml midazolam (10mg/2ml) = 2ml hyoscine butylbromide (400mcg/1ml) = 1.5ml Total volume = 9.5ml. Make up the volume in a 20ml syringe to length 48mm. Set the rate of the driver for 2mm/hr.

7. 2mg x 40mg = 80mg. Administer 2ml or 2 ampoules.

8. 0.8ml

9. Correct amount would be 25ml. Your colleague is incorrect. You need to follow the procedure in your clinical area for near-miss drug errors.

10. 1.5ml

11. 2 tablets

12. Administer 30mg for one-sixth. Administer 0.6ml.

13. 2 puffs

14. 800 mcg

15. 0.8mg

16. 25ml

17. 0.6ml

18. morphine sulphate (60mg/ml) = 1ml midazolam (10mg/2ml) = 2ml metoclopramide (5mg/ml) = 2ml Total volume = 5ml. Make up volume with water for injection to 48mm length in a 10ml syringe and set driver for 2mm/hr.

19. 0.8ml

20. 2 vials

Assessment 9

1. 2.5ml

2. 100mg x 1.8kg = 180mg total daily dose. Divide by 2 to get 90mg twice daily.

3. Add 5ml – 0.4ml (displacement volume) = 4.6ml to make solution of 600mg/5ml. Administer 2ml.

4. 10 dpm (rounding down from 10.4)

5. 154mcg x 12.kg = 1848mcg. Convert to milligrams = 1.848mg. Divide this by 7.7mg to get 0.24ml. Administer 0.24ml.

6. 2.5ml

7. Convert 1mg to micrograms = 1000mcg. Administer 0.24ml.

8. 80mg x 8.6kg = 688mg

9. 1g =1000mg. Administer 6.88ml.

10. 5ml

11. 1 suppository

12. 200mg x 4.9kg = 980mg total dose and 245mg four times a day. Add 2ml – 0.2ml (displacement volume) = 1.8ml to make a solution of 250mg/2ml. Administer 1.96ml.

13. 4mg x 16.8kg = 67.2mg. Administer 4.48ml.

14. 50ml/hr

15. 6ml

16. 30mg x 1.9kg = 57mg

17. 150mcg x 1.2kg = 180mcg. Convert 1mg to micrograms to get 1000/ml. Administer 0.18ml.

18. 0.8mg = 800mg and 200mg four times a day. Administer 10ml each dose.

19. 5mg x 10.2kg = 51mg total dose and 25.5mg twice daily. You should administer 4.25ml. Your colleague is incorrect and you will need to follow the procedure in your clinical area for near-miss drug errors.

20. 800mcg x 38kg = 30400mcg = 30.4mg

Assessment 10

1. 3 vials

2. 3 tablets

3. Should administer 1.5ml so, yes, your colleague is correct.

4. 500ml/hr

5. 125ml/hr

6. 40g glucose and 1.8g sodium chloride

7. Adrenaline 1:1000 = 1mg:1000ml = 1000mg:1000ml = 1mg:1ml. You need to prepare 0.5ml.

8. 500mcg x 46.8kg = 23 400mcg = 23.4mg. Infusion rate needs to be 23.4ml/hr (500mg/500ml = 1mg/1ml).

9. Administer 0.75ml heparin. Set rate as 2ml/hr for 24-hour continuous infusion.

10. 9.7mmols/L = 2 units per hour = 2ml/hr

11. morphine sulphate (60mg/1ml) = 3ml
haloperidol (5mg/1ml) = 0.3ml
metoclopramide (5mg/ml) = 2ml
Total volume = 5.3ml. Make up volume to 48mm length. Set a 24-hour driver for 48mm.

12. 28 dpm (rounding up from 27.7')

13. 4 tablets

14. 4 vials

15. 2mg x 86kg = 172mg. Administer 4.3ml.

16. 80mg/50ml = 1.6mg/1ml. 2.8ml/hr = 2.8 x 1.6mg = 4.48mg/hr

17. morphine sulphate(60mg/1ml) = 2ml
midazolam (10mg/ml) = 1ml
hyoscine butylbromide (400mcg/ml) = 1.5ml

Total volume = 4.5ml. Use a 10ml syringe and make volume to 48mm. Set drive to 48mm for a 24-hour syringe driver.

18. 20ml or 2 vials

19. 2mcg x 67.8kg x $^{60}\!/_{80\,000}$ x 50 = 5.085 or 5.1ml/hr (rounding up)

20. 1.2g = 1200mg divided by 4 = 300mg four times a day. You would need to administer 15ml. Your colleague is incorrect and you need to follow the procedure in your area for near-miss drug errors.

Index